Silent Fields

The Growing Cancer Cluster Story

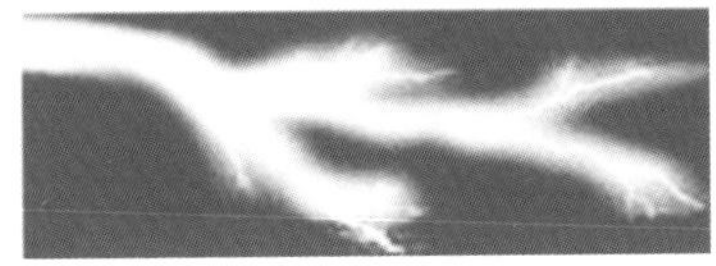

When Electricity Kills....

Silent Fields

The Growing Cancer Cluster Story

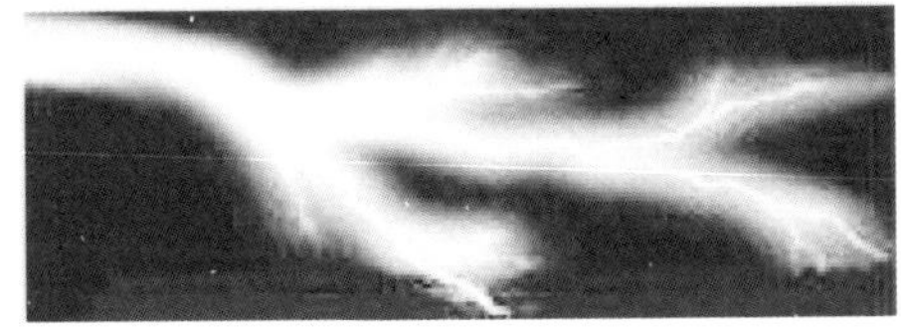

When Electricity Kills....

Donna Fisher

Editor:
Dr Charles Neophytou

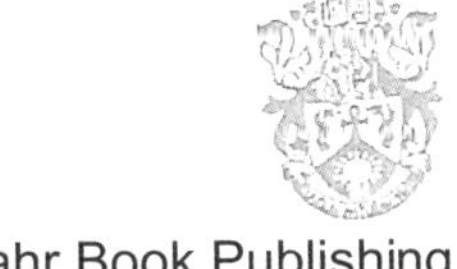

Lindlahr Book Publishing
Charles Neophytou & Associates
Commonwealth of Australia

Lindlahr Book Publishing
Charles Neophytou & Associates
Karragarra Island, Queensland, Australia, 4184

ISBN: 978 0 646 48743 4

A catalogue record for this book is available from the National Library of Australia.

Cover design by Charles Neophytou
Interior design by Linda Neophytou
Printed and bound in Australia by
Kingswood Press Underwood Queensland Australia

Dedicated to all cancer victims and survivors
who bravely face their monster.

*"All the world's a stage and all the men and women are
merely players, they have their exits and entrances, and
one man in his time plays many parts….."*

Shakespeare

Contents

Foreword

$\mathcal{B}$y Lyn Allison

Electricity is something that we have very much taken for granted for the past 100 years. Culminating in the facilitation of a global communications infrastructure involving thousands of mobile phone antennas and satellites, our lives have been revolutionised both personally and professionally. Indeed, it is hard in 2007 to imagine how we ever coped without our mobiles, computers and the internct.

Nevertheless, ten years ago it was brought to my attention by campaigners and scientists around the country that we were taking this huge increase in electromagnetic radiation for granted at a cost. The evidence for a wide range of adverse health effects as a result of exposure to low level electromagnetic fields and other aspects of electromagnetic radiation – technically known as non-thermal effects – led me to instigate a Senate Inquiry in 1998 (on RF EMF), which reported in May 2001.

At this inquiry scientists, electrical engineers and affected individuals from around the world testified that non-thermal effects can – and do cause conditions and illnesses ranging from the mild to the fatal: headaches, memory loss, obesity, arthritis, Alzheimer's, cancer and leukaemia to name but a few. Possible mechanisms included the permeability of the blood brain barrier, calcium ion efflux and the alteration of gene behaviour.

Dr Neil Cherry analysed hundreds of studies done over five decades, which revealed that the science in this area shows a connection between adverse health effects and low-level exposure from either communications infrastructure or substations and powerlines.

Complicating the issue is the fact that electricity in all its forms is highly volatile, and does not easily lend it to being pinned down by current scientific methodologies. This fact is regularly exploited by industry groups, who regularly demand replications of positive studies, which are often hard to produce as results are easily altered by the subtlest changes to the protocol and assay technique. This is over and above the methods of interpreting the data!

Differences of opinion between independent scientists and government and industry bodies in Australia have left some concerned that both the Electromagnetic Radiation (EMR) and Extremely Low Frequency (ELF) exposure standards have not been adequately adjusted to reflect the adverse health effects caused by the low levels that have been indicated by some studies. The new standard is due to be finalised later this year.

Given that the World Health Organisation has classified low-level EMR and ELF as a Class 2B carcinogen I can only assume that this standard has not been produced to protect the public but to the interests of the industries involved.

This book is an excellent snapshot of the issues, the science, and the difficulties and trials facing anyone who attempts to assert their rights to not only create a safe and healthy home and work environment, but also to have their concerns recognised by the legal system and the government.

Lyn Allison (former senator)
Melbourne, 2007

Acknowledgements

*I*t is with sincere thanks that I acknowledge the contributions of:

- Mr Alexander (Sandy) Doull, whose decision to support our case, contributed to delivering the landmark achievement

- The late Professor Ross Adey MD, well known EMF veteran also for his recommendation that that I read *The Melatonin Hypothesis: Breast Cancer and Use of Electric Power* which fed my quest to find out more, particularly on the issue of breast cancer

- The late Associate Professor Neil Cherry, MD PhD

- Professor Denis Henshaw of H H Wills Physics Laboratory, University of Bristol, Britain, United Kingdom

- Associate Professor Magda Havas BSc PhD, Environmental and Research Studies, Trent University, Canada

- Louis Slesin, PhD, Editor of *Microwave News*, New York, United States of America

- Ms Cindy Sage MA, Sage Associates, California, United States of America

- Mr Don Maisch, EMFacts Consultancy, Tasmania, Australia

- Ms Lyn McLean, *EMR and Health*, Sydney, Australia

- Dr Maximilian Moser, Institute of Noninvasive Diagnosis, Joanneum Research, Franz-Pichler Strasse 30, A-8160 Weiz, Austria for handing me the graph on breast cancer risk used in Appendix F.

who were all very generous with their time and willing to answer our group's many questions in the lead-up to the court case and in the writing of this book.

Our small group consisted of Cheryl and Jim Kerr, Jenny and Greg Cadwallader, my husband Cameron and I. Mitch Wagner, David

Turner, Gerard Walters and environmentalist Ted Fensom were also against the sub-station proposal.

I would like to extend special thanks to Cheryl and Jim Kerr and Jenny and Greg Cadwallader. I would also like to emphasise their role in helping to achieve the landmark court decision and their support in the writing of this book. It was the equally strong conviction of our three families that helped us through the periods when we thought we had run out of all avenues to pursue our stand.

Finally, it is the work of the many scientists who have dedicated years of research in this area that has resulted in the writing of this book. I hope that I have done justice to their research and their painstaking endeavours to bring attention to the most important health issue of our times.

This story is about a battle between a small group of people living along an urban street in Tanah Merah, a suburb in Logan City on the outskirts of Brisbane, Queensland and one of the largest public companies in Queensland, Energex.

It started as a battle over the location of an urban power sub-station. The community saw the sub-station as a serious threat to the health of members of the community, and especially its children.

But it's a big ask for a handful of people to take on a large utility, especially when we had limited understanding of the technical and scientific language.

One

$\mathcal{D}$aybreak is normally sudden and swift in Queensland, but on this day it was breaking gently. Cued by the dawn light, birdsong began. It was a promise of a gorgeous day as the dawn lit up the sky and the new day was beginning. At first the melodious and somewhat poignant song of the magpie together with the joyous laughter of the kookaburra soon blended into the rich birdsong flooding the air. I was lying in bed on this morning savouring the sweetest sounds when my mind was brought to fuller consciousness by the sharp "karri-karrik-karrik" and "kek-kekkekekeke" rapid burst of the masked lapwing plover for the purpose of protecting their young and communicating danger Now it was wake up time for me ……..mother's work is never done, children to be fed and prepared for school, breakfast for mum and dad and later …….. much later Donna Fisher, writer and erstwhile little warrior turns her attention to everyday living and to do battle with a multi-national company that is at the moment more important than life itself. Forget now the zealous cries of the Australian pink and grey galah blasting away at my home at Tanah Merah……it's time to go, go, go.

Just for a split second to a minute I glance sideways across the bed to the figure of my husband Cameron who is still peacefully sleeping on despite the machine gun rattle of the plover. Cameron a giant of a man is a constant source of support in all my battles in life over the last 20 years. Currently he is supporting my social activation and as a soul-mate is encouraging me to make discovery of the facts surrounding so-called "dirty" electricity. At first Cameron was a little uncertain about just how electricity could be a problem to the health and welfare of its users and later I was to discover in most people that I encountered this uncertainty about electricity being a problem. This included so called "authorities" in the know, so to speak. Cameron was not one to simply go into denial about so-called problemed electricity. His enquiries soon led him to understand the hazards of "dirty" electricity.

I had been engaged in other projects and studies that were fulfilling requirements for a thesis study, the subject being the role that women played in civilization throughout the ages. I was actively engaged in studies of Transpersonal Philosophy and I was also playing a leading role in management of our family's commercial business and at the same time enjoying the rearing of our three children. Little did I know that things were going to change in the ole corral. The change started on July 24th 2006 to be exact. This was when I became aware of the so-called breast cancer cluster at the ABC's Television Studios in the suburb of Toowong. It was not news to me. As many other women, I am aware that breast cancer is a concern and over the years I have heard that breast cancer, once a disease of the western world was fast becoming a global concern. Like most other women I thought about what caused cancer but not really in depth. I suppose that is the case for all of us. It is only really when those close to us are afflicted by some disease that we sit up and take notice. It is a pity this happens but that is how it is – only when we or those closest to us are touched by such tragic occurrences that we build up both empathy and knowledge to understand that we could be the next victim. No doubt that is the way of the selfish gene.

I'll never forget that day in July 2006. Something then was telling me to find out more about cancer clusters. I still don't know what that "something" was but I started my inquiry in the most logical way – research. My research came easily to me as I understood the logic of research. Maths and logic have always been my strong points. Then at the ABC Studios the breast cancer cluster count stood at 12 (it is now at 17 and still climbing) – 12 women with breast cancer and all who worked at the studio! What was going on? I got hold of an instrument – a gaussmeter (by now very familiar to me), after finding out how to measure magnetic fields. I also remember thinking to myself: "Donna, you're becoming a proper little "scientist" without a degree – but with lots of guts"......(I was greatly inspired by an intensive two day Leadership course I attended in Perth, Western Australia called "The Way of the Stone"). Among other things the course taught that in life we are all dealt a certain hand and where we find ourselves on a "board" is where we have to be the best and give our all to survive and thrive. The course fashioned a drafting board broken up in squares showing situations. By throwing a stone onto the board each person had to explain how they would be the "best stone" (warrior) they could be by improvising, adapting, surviving to thrive in each situation. This action had to be done with great honour for this is the Way of the Warrior nothing above honour. So here I am now.....a stone (warrior) in Queensland where "dirty" electricity is causing cancer and other diseases, threatening the lives of many people. As arrogant as it sounds I have a role to play in creating awareness of cancer clusters – and this I will do.

On the 26th July 2006 I went to the ABC site 25 minutes from my home and measured the fields on the footpath of the premises. I measured fields of 26mG with my gaussmeter. Please note that the building was very close to the footpath.

I rang Channel 9 TV and spoke to Lexie Hamilton-Smith who advised me of the staff reference committee for the ABC dilemma. Ian Eckersley, Lisa Backhouse and Nadia Farhar were on this committee. She stated Nadia Farhar nearly died from breast cancer. I rang Nadia and gave her brief details and she suggested I call a Professor Armstrong. I also asked if it was possible to have someone on staff take in a small appliance to take some measurements but I did not make much progress here. I sent her some information on electromagnetic radiation which I had researched.

A few weeks later I once again took measurements on the footpath but went onto the premises against the wall and the measurement was 11.4mG. I was advised by the security guard to leave the premises. When I went back to try and see Nadia I noticed they had put a black fence around the area where I measured. I tried to contact her again but could never get on to her. I arrived at the studios one day to try and see her but was advised by the security guard that she was not there. I took measurements while I was on the premises – the security guard's office was on the premises. The measurements changed from 9 – 14mG.

I went back several times between July 2006 and December 2006 and the readings were always around 9 – 14mG. I also hired another gaussmeter to check my measurements.

By now and through inquires with scientists in the field and with experts both for and against, it became clear that electromagnetic radiation could even in modest doses turn some healthy people into cancer victims. These are invisible and silent fields with murder in mind.

At this stage I decided there was a story to tell especially about when Energex – the giant energy company was going to locate an urban power sub-station in my street even though they did not know the extent of electromagnetic radiation and its relationship to breast cancer and childhood leukaemia. There is no doubt this is when the selfish gene kicked in, and thank goodness it did, for this together with the warrior ideal which I had learnt about in Perth spurred me into action. It has been said by many friends and foe alike that it was here that the battle started and in many ways this book is the story of intrigue and many battles within battles.

Essentially therefore in the onset this story begins with the first battle – a battle between a small group of people living along an urban street in Tanah Merah, a suburb in Logan City on the outskirts of Brisbane, Queensland and one of the largest public companies in Queensland, Energex.

It started as a dispute over the location of an urban power sub-station and up-graded powerlines. The community saw the sub-station as a serious threat to the health of members of the community, and especially its children.

But it's a big ask for a handful of people to take on a large utility, especially when we had limited understanding of the technical and scientific language but as the old adage states "power to the people" and that is just what happened…… we improvised, we adapted and with lots of sweat and tears won the day, but only the day. There is still a lot to do before we can claim victory as the health of many healthy people is still under threat from "dirty" electricity.

As most of us already know invisible and usually silent fields permeate our environment. They emanate from a variety of sources including: powerlines, sub-stations, electronic equipment and electrical appliances. As a result of the landmark court case in the Planning and Environment Court in November 2001 between Energex, the Logan City Council and the Sewell Road resident group, other communities have sought information on the invisible fields that we are exposed to every day. Many believe as I do that some of the fields are toxic and can be linked to breast cancer in more than a tenuous way. Over the past 3 years I have also alerted media outlets but too often the subject is regarded as too complicated and not fully taken up. Yet this very important health issue is a newer language that we must all understand. Besides, if we are right, surely the authorities should be more careful. Despite this confidence in the efficacy of public infrastructure companies, there are serious and mounting concerns by world leading scientists about the impact on people's health of exposure to man-made radiation. 'Sick Building Syndrome' is now being given more attention. In July 2006, seven cases of brain tumours at the RMIT University in Victoria came to my attention. At the same time the University of NSW on its Kensington campus is investigating a possible cancer cluster after staff expressed concerns about the high incidence of the disease among those working in a building. Further incidence of cancers at a school in Hobart and so too at Milpera State School in Queensland have also just come to attention as well as staff also raising concern at an electronics energy division near Sydney. These instances are but a few of the many excessive cancer cases being linked to man-made fields around the world.

Also, in July 2006 I was alerted to the high incidence of breast cancer in women who worked at the ABC TV studios in Toowong, Queensland, Australia. My experience in the court case and research strongly suggested that the problem at the ABC TV studios would include exposure to electromagnetic fields (EMF), as every case was breast cancer. From 1994 until late 2007, seventeen staff who worked in a particular area at this site have been diagnosed with breast cancer. I had seen first-hand how these investigations were conducted and I assert they're not conducted correctly.

The investigation would be lengthy and cumbersome, panels would be set up for both sides, and no workplace factor found that could explain the unusual collection of disease.

In December 2006 an independent panel for the ABC TV studios estimated that there was a one in a million probability that chance was involved. The statistical findings suggested that women working at this location were up to eleven times more likely to get breast cancer than the general population. A breast cancer cluster was reported. As all other factors had been discounted, the problem was deemed to be work-place related.

Meanwhile, a prominent health specialist and researcher at Sydney University, Professor Bruce Armstrong led the investigation which examined ten of the breast cancer cases at the ABC. He recorded that the ABC had no option other than to abandon the site yet the many experts engaged to determine the problem found no cause. A large proportion of staff left immediately on 21 December 2006. Staff members have been relocated. Professor Armstrong believes it is reasonable to expect there will be more cases which could possibly persist for up to five years. I believe it will be more like ten years.

"Dirty" electricity has more than just a tenuous link to cancer. In fact this breast cancer cluster at the ABC is what prompted the writing of this book. This book will raise awareness to the hazards being associated with powerlines, sub-stations and the inadequate planning that allows homes to be built in close proximity to electrical power systems. Also of concern is inadequate planning that can result in hazardous work-places.

There will be, but shouldn't be, prolonged suffering yet more people will suffer health-wise before change occurs. In July 2007 Concord hospital in Sydney revealed it had launched a preliminary investigation in May 2007 after five female workers were diagnosed with breast cancer between 2001 and 2006 and who had worked in a limited area of the hospital. Efforts are now being made to establish how many more cases there have been in current and past staff (some are understood to have died) as the figure is rising. However, by expediting awareness of potential health risks the attendant potential for litigation (which has the potential to dwarf the asbestos experience) may be minimized.

There is hope when the powerful ACTU (Australian Council of Trade Unions) commences collating information on work-place cancer clusters around Australia.

The fields we are exposed to emanate from:

- powerlines (which establishes the ambient background fields that permeate our homes and workplaces) and,

- wiring in buildings and electrical appliances and equipment (such as hairdryers, alarm clocks, refrigerators, microwaves, computers, photo-developing machines, hospital equipment, baby monitors, humidicribs, etc.).

The fields emitted from these sources are extremely low frequency electromagnetic fields. ELF EMF is the abbreviation most commonly used.

The risks most commonly associated with exposures have included:

- leukaemia – especially in children
- brain tumours
- breast cancers
- Lou Gehrig's disease

All these diseases are increasing. Cancer clusters associated with these fields are becoming more apparent with more than just a tenuous link to breast cancer. Authorities around the world are beginning to adopt guidelines, albeit slowly, to protect the public from their cancer-causing effects. However their responses are limited to discussion groups, lots of conferences, much consulting and bewildering muddle – just not good enough when so much is at stake.

Two

"*D*o substations pose health risks?

International research has concluded that there is insufficient evidence to come to a firm conclusion regarding possible health effects from exposure to power frequency electric and magnetic fields".

This paragraph in the two-page letter from our electricity supplier, Energex, alarmed our small group in our street in 1999. This paragraph was the catalyst that started my close neighbours and myself on a long and involved fight against the proposal to locate a new sub-station and powerlines very close to our homes.

Our beautiful street, Sewell Road, Tanah Merah, Queensland, is administered by Logan City Council. The street with a population of young children and parents living on acreages until then had been virtually untouched by the expansion of the city. Our quiet and relaxed lifestyle was about to change.

Greg Cadwallader, the taxi driver who lived across from my house and two blocks of land up from the proposed sub-station site had been besieged by cancer. Jenny, a mother, would subsequently suffer breast cancer. They had powerlines running within 7 metres from their bedroom until they were removed. My next-door neighbours, Jim, a commercial artist and Cheryl, a school teacher, were very concerned as the proposed sub-station was to be directly across the narrow street from their home. Cheryl had lived next door to a sub-station in her childhood. Her father had died of a brain tumour. Two other neighbours to that sub-station had also died from brain tumours.

Cameron, the Managing Director of a Transport Company and myself, a mother, director and mature age student studying feminist principles in the modern world, lived next-door to the Kerr's.

We were a normal, small neighbourhood group that would be transformed into a community force determined to challenge one of the most powerful public sector companies in Queensland.

As a group we began reviewing the research into the impact of sub-stations. As we contacted those with experience we grew increasingly concerned about the fields that emanated from sub-stations and powerlines. Something seemed terribly wrong and whatever it was, it was about to be directly imposed on us. We also came to understand that the proposed sub-station was only one part of the system that was to be upgraded and that other lines could expose more people in the community to higher levels of these fields than those that previously existed.

Our small group found it was vital to learn a technical language that was quite foreign to us. What were these fields from powerlines? The key terms for our research were: **magnetic fields** and **electromagnetic fields**.

As a group we began the vital though laborious investigation not knowing exactly what these fields were. It was almost back to school for us to find out the abc's of electricity. Up until now we hadn't cared much about how the light sub-stations worked. Electric and magnetic fields are produced wherever electricity is generated, transmitted or used. They are odourless, invisible and most often, silent. Together these fields are termed 'electromagnetic fields' (EMF). EMF are electromagnetic fields that emanate from powerlines, sub-stations, wiring in buildings and electrical appliances and equipment (i.e., hairdryers, alarm clocks, microwaves, computers, photo-developing machines, hospital equipment, humidicribs, etc.).

These fields are referred to as extremely low frequency (ELF) fields. **ELF EMF** is the most common abbreviation for extremely low frequency electromagnetic fields. (ELF on its own or EMF on its own are sometimes used).

The power system is an alternating system, operating at 50 cycles per second, i.e., it has a frequency of 50 Hertz (Hz) in Europe, Australia and many other countries. In the United States, Canada and parts of Japan, the AC frequency is 60 Hz.

Just by way of simple logic: Electric fields are produced by voltage. The strength of the electric field depends on the voltage and is present in any live wire even when electricity is not being used. Electric fields are measured in volts/metres (V/m).

Electric currents produce magnetic fields – the more current the more intense the field. The magnetic field drops off rapidly with increasing distance from the source.

IMPORTANT

Magnetic fields are measured in milliGauss (mG), for example, 1mG, 2mG, 3mG, 4mG. We discovered that the difference between a measurement of 1mG, 2mG, 3mG and 4mG and so on could have enormous implications on our health. This then is the crux – measurements must be taken to establish when exactly electricity kills.

Further afield in the USA epidemiologist Dr Nancy Wertheimer and electrical engineer Ed Leeper in Denver, Colorado, conducted a study in 1979 that brought worldwide attention to the link between EMF and childhood leukaemia. Wertheimer and Leeper noticed in their hotly debated epidemiological research that children who were twice or three times as likely to have leukaemia, tended to live in homes in the Denver area close to powerlines and transformers. Their results were published in a scientific paper, and found an increased incidence of childhood leukaemia, lymphomas and nervous system tumours for children.

(Refer Nancy Wertheimer, Ed Leeper; *Electrical Wiring Configurations and Childhood Cancer*; American Journal of Epidemiology, Vol. 109 (3): 273-284, 1979).

Their results had an immediate effect as in response to public opposition to the construction of new high voltage lines, the electrical industry convened an expert panel of eminent and conservative medical scientists. Included in this panel was Professor David Carpenter from the New York University Department of Public Health and Dr David Savitz, one of America's most respected epidemiologists.

Carpenter's original scepticism was overturned when the Wertheimer and Leeper study, originally heavily criticised as flawed, was extended and improved. It confirmed a significantly increased risk of leukaemias. Dr David Savitz reported that twenty percent of childhood cancers were attributable to exposure at 3 milliGauss.

(Refer Savitz, *et al.*; *Case-control Study of Childhood Cancer and Exposure to 60-Hz Magnetic Fields*; American Journal of Epidemiology, Vol 128, No. 1, 1988).

Nancy Wertheimer and Ed Leeper then conducted a study of adult cancer risk and their results showed that adults aged below 55 years, living long-term in residences permeated by magnetic fields of 3mG and greater, had significantly higher rates of four types of cancer due to their close proximity to high current carrying electrical power lines. These were cancers of the nervous system, uterus, breast and lymphomas.

(Refer Wertheimer N, Leeper, E, *Adult cancer related to electrical wires near the home.* Int J Epidemiol. 1982; 11:345-55).

The current guidelines in Australia, as in most other countries (with some countries even higher), allow constant exposure to 1000mG.

Since the now-famous Wertheimer and Leeper study extensive epidemiological research into the human health effects of extremely low frequency electromagnetic fields has been conducted.

Throughout the world residential and occupational studies have repeatedly found associations with a range of diseases, which include:

- leukaemia
- tumours of the brain and central nervous system
- breast cancers for both males and females
- increased risks of Alzheimer's and Lou Gehrig's disease

Many research centres are beginning to work on identifying credible standards although most countries have not yet addressed the issue of appropriate standards to set for 'potential' hazardous effects from these fields. A scientific working party of the US National Radiation Measurement and Protection Commission assessed all the available health effects literature up to 1996. Finding the 1000mG exposure guideline incapable of protecting the population against the risk of cancers, it proposed a strategy based on the radiation safety principle of keeping human exposures as low as reasonably achievable. The 'As Low As Reasonably Achievable Approach' (ALARA) was an immediate move to 10mG and a scheduled reduction over ten years to 2mG. This has yet to be implemented.

In 1999 a Swiss Government Ordinance introduced a human exposure standard of 10mG for magnetic field exposures for new installations. **This was a huge drop from 1000mG.**

Later in 1999 two studies were published that changed the way the risk of cancer from powerlines would be understood. Findings from previous studies were combined and pooled and a new, more powerful analysis (meta-analysis) was run on the cancer data. These worldwide studies by Greenland *et al.* 2000 (which included 15 studies) and Ahlbom *et al.* 2000 (which included 9 of the individual studies) confirmed there is an increased leukaemia risk in children.

Clearly, we had enough facts to make a stand against the sub-station proposal.

Deeply concerned by what further research was revealing our small group contacted Pam Parker our local councillor from the Logan City Council. Pam was also concerned, simply stating: "I am with you all the way".

Our small group lobbied people in the street to support our cause. Many residents were too busy to become actively involved but all were uneasy. Everyone had a disturbing story to tell about powerlines or sub-stations: excessive cases of cancer in humans, birds behaving strangely, cows supplying less milk or horses delivering stillborn foals. In fact, any species living close to powerlines and sub-stations seemed to be affected. We began social activation progress. Leaflets were sent out and we urged people to write letters against having a sub-station in our street.

Shortly after, our group was invited to a meeting at the Logan City Council chambers with council staff and five men from Energex. At this meeting we submitted our concerns.

We discussed how the Wertheimer and Leeper study had brought worldwide attention to the fields from powerlines and sub-stations and that many other countries had since conducted their own studies. We spoke about Paul Brodeur's book *The Great Power-Line Cover-up* and the attention bought to a particular street where a sub-station was close to houses and how serious disease had presented. (Meadow Street, Connecticut in the United States had only nine houses yet seven adults and children had been stricken with cancer).

We bought attention to the Swedes who operate on the presumption that the fields from powerlines are carcinogenic. They had come to this conclusion when medical research conducted in co-operation with the electrical utility completed a twenty-five year study (1960-1985), linking every childhood leukaemia case with measurements of the fields at the homes and with electrical utility power load records. This study concluded that childhood leukaemia was four times greater where children lived in a 300nT (3mG) field or greater and three times greater when living in a 200nT (2mG) fields. *SWEDES — 1960-1985*

We informed the council that in Russia itself restrictions were in place to limit human exposure to these fields and the Swedish Government was supporting prudent avoidance measures by setting boundaries to protect their citizens.

We submitted that we pay the electricity companies and yet magnetic and electric fields, which we now considered a toxic agent, are permeating our environment.

We then repeated what was stated in the first correspondence from Energex in 1999:

> "Do substations pose health risks?
>
> International research has concluded that there is insufficient evidence to come to a firm conclusion regarding possible health effects from exposure to power frequency electric and magnetic fields".

In conclusion we stated: "It is not for those who emit these fields as a by-product who should have the benefit of the doubt but rather those who are exposed to its 'potentially' deadly outcome".

Energex, a State Government owned corporation, is one of Australia's largest and fastest-growing organisations with more than 3800 staff working in a range of roles to supply electricity to a population of around 2.7 million people in south-east Queensland. A top 100 Australian company with $6.6 billion in total assets, Energex has more than 80 years industry experience and describes itself as "one of the most respected companies in the country recently winning awards for customer communications, its strong environmental focus and community safety".

The directors are appointed by the Governor in Council in accordance with the provisions of the Government Owned Corporations Act 1993.

Energex's distribution area of 25,000 square kilometres includes more than 50,000 km of underground and overhead electricity lines and cables, over half a million power poles, some 43,000 transformers and more than 290,000 street lights. The company's web-site says the Board monitors environmental and safety performance on a continuing basis, and has systems in place to review controls and ensure compliance with laws and ethical behaviour. In this case Energex stated the fields would be well below the Australian guideline of 1000mG.

Like people who have challenged the power of cigarette companies, we felt that trying to negotiate with the energy companies would not be fruitful. Those closest to the proposed site wanted to leave the street. We were concerned about the consequences to our health. We asked that our homes be bought out but compensation was not seen as necessary. Energex simply stated that the sub-station had to go ahead. The Sewell Road community disagreed. I held a meeting with the Mayor of Logan City Council, Cr John Freeman.

Mayor Freeman wanted the magnetic field information further explained. He, like all of us, sought a clearer understanding of this new language which was incomprehensible jargon to ordinary citizens despite the fact that powerlines had been a contentious issue for decades. In fact we discovered that the whole EMF issue is one of the most important public health issues of our times. This is another reason for writing this book.

After looking at the issue more closely, council rejected the planning application by Energex.

Some months later Energex again applied for permission to build the sub-station. As a concession to the community it was now proposed to put it on the block of land next door to the original block. This was one block further away but to our group still too close to residential houses. Once again we fought back with letters to council.

Cr Pam Parker once again joined our fight. Once again council rejected the Energex application. We were all delighted, our faith in 'people power' justified. This had been a lengthy process and we were happy to get on with our busy lives but our peace of mind was to be short lived. Energex decided to appeal against council's rejection of the second sub-station site proposal.

In January 2001 Energex wrote to citizens who had sent letters opposing the second sub-station site notifying that we would be co-respondents in a court case to be held in the Planning and Environment Court, Brisbane. Our small group was obliged to fight, to put up or shut up. Unfortunately none of us had experience in this kind of law so a new learning curve had to begin.

The court case was listed as Energex Limited versus Logan City Council and Co-respondents. Even though council also opposed the sub-station proposal the community group was obliged to prepare a separate case and retain our own expert witnesses.

After consultations with various solicitors, we realised that winning the case was going to be difficult as EMF and adverse health effects had not been the central issue in any court case in Australia.

Our group decided to seek help from the State Government. On visiting the Department of Energy in Brisbane we were informed that as the issue was already in the legal system the Government could not interfere.

There was one particular issue in this case that was most concerning. In one of their letters to our street, Energex had stated: "Energex abides by the current interim guidelines on limits of exposure to 50/60 Hz and magnetic fields by the National Health and Medical Research Council".

We again referred back to previous Energex correspondence that stated:

> "No prescriptive standards currently exist to limit the level of EMF to which the general public may be exposed in their everyday lives, however the Australian National Health and Medical Research Council (NHMRC) has published exposure guidelines, viz, interim guidelines on limits of exposure to 50/60Hz electric and magnetic fields (1989). These are based on established or predicted effects and also on publications of the International Non-ionising Radiation Association (under the auspices of the World Health Organisation).
>
> The guideline limit for continuous public exposure in this document is 1000mG for magnetic fields. The corresponding limit for electric fields is 5 kV/m. For the Tanah Merah sub-station, electric and magnetic field strengths resulting from the equipment contained therein are within the guidelines at any distance."

These two sentences stood out:-

> No prescriptive standards currently exist to limit the level of EMF to which the general public may be exposed in their everyday lives.

> The guideline limit for continuous public exposure in this document is 1000mG for magnetic fields.

The research was indicating 4mG and even 2mG was a problem. How was this connected to the 1000mG guideline in place? What was going on?

The published evidence of at least an association between powerlines and childhood cancer seemed to be substantial and persuasive. In our opinion, this evidence should not be ignored.

Then on March 6, 2001 an advisory group of Britain's National Radiological Protection Board (NRPB) released the 'Doll Report'. This study was important, as it was the first official statement from a major health organization in the United Kingdom.

The 'Doll Report' found 4mG was the level at which a doubling of childhood leukaemia risk occurred often enough to be significant. This was nowhere near 1000mG.

The man who made this story so newsworthy was the chairman of the NRPB's advisory group, Sir Richard Doll, the famous epidemiologist who was knighted for identifying the association between smoking and lung-cancer in the 1950s. It was reported that Doll was originally sceptical of the findings of possible hazards from powerlines.

In a signed letter from Energex, dated 21 March 2001, in response to one of our letters, Energex stated: "There is, however, some epidemiological evidence that prolonged exposure to higher levels of ELF magnetic fields is associated with a small risk of leukaemia in children". What they did not state was that there were also many studies showing adults at risk.

Our situation was looking pretty dismal yet my visit to a woman named Angie, who previously worked at the Capalaba Post Office, Brisbane, was a compelling reminder of the importance of the battle we were now engaged in. Angie was one of fifty-three people who had developed serious or fatal diseases at this work site.

A sub-station was built close to the Post Office on the next door property.

A signed letter from the Queensland Premier's Chief of Staff dated 24 September 2001, in regard to the Capalaba Post Office situation, stated that there was no scientific evidence to conclude that the causes of illnesses by former staff were linked. Key findings included:

- The most likely explanation for the various diseases among current and former staff is that their occurrence is a coincidence;
- There is no workplace factor that could explain the unusual collection of diseases and health complaints.

We realised this was a typical response to concerned communities around the world, communities which were forced to fight through the legal system. Then we discovered that elevated electromagnetic fields were also being associated with an increased incidence of male breast cancer, a rare form of the disease. There was an incidence overseas where three men had contracted breast cancer in the same office and, as this occurrence was particularly bizarre, two of them were also being forced to fight through the legal system.

There was no chance of sorting this out sensibly through mediation or some other conflict resolution modality. I thought that with Energex it was the adversarial system where they hoped to crush the little people – the aussie battlers. That was the way of this industry and we were all wondering how our small group could successfully fight against this proposal when Cr Pam Parker mentioned that a day long conference was to be held at the Chancellor on the Park in Brisbane, not long before our court case. Although it was for the telecommunications industry we decided it might provide interesting insights for our community group.

They were discussing the way telecommunications equipment emitted electromagnetic radiation, focusing on RF EMF (RFR – radio frequency radiation – mobile phone towers) rather than ELF EMF (Refer to Appendix B).

The audience was packed with employees from different firms and from councils who were being advised that there was basically nothing wrong with mobile phone towers and that the public was more interested in how these towers looked near their homes and how these towers affected their real estate prices. It was being intimated that people were not really concerned about their health and we knew who had started these rumours.

We also discarded Michael Bangay's assertions, a technical officer with the Australian Radiation Protection and Nuclear Safety Agency (ARPANSA) who was one of the keynote speakers at this meeting. The impact of the silent fields on human health was discounted with the "so-called" expert's words I will always remember: "There is a slight leukaemia risk; these fields affect only a few children in every 100,000".

Even a tenuous link to leukaemia was not and is not trivial as most mothers and others would agree.

On being asked about the connection between powerlines and childhood leukaemia, Michael Bangay referred to a Neil Cherry who had come to Australia to testify.

There was a suggestion of triumphalism in the ensuing discussion and it became apparent from the meeting that this Dr Cherry was struggling to have his view accepted in Australia. Among other things, Dr Cherry's use of the word 'genotoxic' (directly damages the precious genetic material of cells) in regard to these fields was ridiculed.

To the insiders of the industry, Dr Cherry was an outsider to be defeated.

Their rejection of his views was too glib in our opinion so we decided to discover why he, of the hundreds of scientists working on this issue, had been singled out for attention. An unpopular expert, no doubt!

Associate Professor Neil Cherry of New Zealand gave evidence to an Australian Senate Enquiry in 1998. Bangay was not enthusiastic about the views of Professor Cherry. We had not previously heard of Neil Cherry so the reference gave us an important lead.

It became important to establish whether Dr Cherry was a sound and credible authority. We contacted Blake B. Levitt (author of *Electromagnetic Fields: A consumer's guide to the issues and how to protect ourselves*) who recommended we contact Neil Cherry and Cindy Sage of Sage Associates – EMF consultants – in California, the United States. Cindy Sage commended his work directing us to Associate Professor Neil Cherry in New Zealand. Her reference was confirmed by Don Maisch of Emfacts Consultancy in Australia and led to Professor Denis Henshaw in the United Kingdom, Louis Slesin PhD in the United States, and Sandy Doull in Australia.

Neil Cherry was an Associate Professor of Environmental Health at Lincoln University in New Zealand. Educated in physics he had travelled the world, visiting universities and laboratories collecting published papers, analysing studies and discussing findings with original researchers. Acknowledged as the first scientist to compile and analyze the scientific evidence showing how ELF EMF (and RF EMF) interacts with biology, he made it his mission to educate policymakers and citizens worldwide over the relatively short time he devoted himself to this work, during the last 9 years of his life. He also spoke to many different governments and the European Parliamentary Conference.

To help us understand the EMF health issue, Neil Cherry gave our group a report that he had prepared for a primary school in Florida which was opposing an unacceptably close placement of a sub-station. This report summarised the whole EMF issue producing data from around 40 epidemiological studies that showed a dose-response relationship between exposures and disease.

Our concerns were heightened. Cherry reported that Ramot and McGrath (1982) found a dramatic shift from childhood lymphoma to leukaemia (ALL) that occurred in the Arab population in the Gaza Strip after the introduction of electric power reticulation to homes.

The report also referred to the work of S. Milham and E.M. Ossiander of the Washington Department of Health, Olympia who concluded that the childhood leukaemia peak of common acute lymphoblastic leukaemia (cALL) was attributable to residential electrification: 75% of all childhood acute lymphoblastic leukaemia and 60% of all childhood leukaemia could be preventable.

(Refer Milham, S and Ossiander, E.M., 2001: *Historical evidence that residential electrification caused the emergence of the childhood leukaemia peak.* Medical Hypotheses 56 (3):1 6).

Milham and Ossiander also stated that as early as 1960 Court Brown and Doll recognised that a new leukaemia agent had been introduced into the UK and the US in the 1920s and 1930s but did not make the connection to electrification. No epidemiological studies had been done to follow up this report.

(Refer Court Brown, W.M., Doll, R. *Leukaemia in childhood and young adult life: Trends in mortality in relation to aetiology.* BMJ 1961; 26:981-988).

Cherry advised that cancer development usually took decades although for very young children the cancer development rate was much faster. This was because the cell cycle of young children is much quicker and their immune system is undeveloped because their melatonin production was low. (The faster the cells duplicate the higher the chance something can go wrong and that a cancer cell may form). Cancer could be initiated *in utero* and that this was likely to be the case for early childhood ALL (acute lymphoblastic leukaemia) and AML (acute myeloid leukaemia). The promotion phase could commence *in utero* and continue after birth if the exposure to the toxic agent continued.

Cherry concluded that ELF EMF did influence the rapid cancer development in children, producing some leukaemia cases in the 1st year of life, with the rate continuing to rise to peak in years 3 to 4.

Professor Henshaw of H H Wills Physics Laboratory, University of Bristol, United Kingdom explained that in 2000 three autonomous regions of Italy introduced strict limits for magnetic field exposures near schools, even more strict than the Swiss. Appearing on the *60 Minutes* television program in Australia on May 27 2001 Professor Henshaw observed that in Sweden and many states in the USA there was a prudent avoidance distance of 150 metres and that there is also the practice of avoiding building houses near high voltage powerlines.

In Sweden where the Government announced that it would act on the presumption that exposure to power frequency electromagnetic fields was a cancer risk, prudent avoidance meant that no new children's facilities were to be built in areas where ambient fields exceeded 2-3mG. The Swedish Government incorporated 2mG as a guideline value in its official prudent avoidance position to assist urban planning.

Louis Slesin PhD, founder and editor of *Microwave News*, New York, had been covering developments in the research into the hazards of exposure to radiation from powerlines and other sources since the 1980s. *Microwave News* presented articles and studies on ELF EMF and RF EMF.

Sandy Doull suggested that we contact Roger Lamb, an electrical engineer. Roger's company was Brunswick Energy & Environmental Services Pty Ltd in Eltham, Victoria. Many private companies working towards reducing the exposure of their employees to these 'silent fields' had engaged the services of Roger Lamb.

It became clear that setting standards for a different measure be the thrust in the future.

We were particularly perplexed about one issue. We could not understand the discrepancy between the 1000mG allowed by Australian standards and government regulation, and the 2mG and 1mG that Cherry believed was still a concern. Indeed Dr Cherry thought it wrong to assume that any level was safe.

"They were different things", explained Roger.

The 1000mG guideline was for the 'gross' effects, that is, 'thermal' effects – a significant change in temperature, such as experienced through electric shocks and burns on the body – immediate.

The authorities operate from the premise that, if these extreme 'acute' effects do not occur, then it is not possible for other effects to occur and human beings are safe at all lower field intensities. The guideline had nothing to do with cancer and the silent fields.

Most of the world authorities and suppliers of electricity did not acknowledge the biological, cancer-causing effects (the low level exposures).

Roger's words: "the 1000mG guideline applies only to the 'gross' effects, not to the more 'subtle' but serious biological effects" was the answer we were looking for. They were never intended to protect people from cancer risks where the process of disease is invisible. The 1000mG guidelines were utterly inadequate and irrelevant to the issues at Sewell Road, Tanah Merah.

It was frightening to discover but not entirely unexpected that the power companies could claim to 'operate within current guidelines' with no liability at all when the guidelines being quoted were irrelevant to the problem. Such was the case with cigarette companies in the past. Just higher the threshold, set a different standard i.e. muddy-the-waters and get the law on your side.

Individuals can be exposed to up to 1000mG yet research was indicating that serious illnesses could arise from repeated exposures to only 2mG.

There is no Federal or State Planning or Health Standards regulating: easement sizes or locations of powerlines in proximity to homes or children's facilities or the location and design of sub-stations and switch-rooms as far as field emissions are concerned.

The court case was scheduled for November 2001 and time was running out. Our small group could not afford an expert witness to lodge a report and appear for us in court. After contacting many solicitors and barristers we could not get anyone to work *pro bono*.

Three

*I*t was back in 1996 when the World Health Organisation (WHO) established the International Electromagnetic Fields Project to address health issues associated with exposure to EMF.

Only a few months before our court case, in June 2001, after more than twenty years of extensive research, there was a major announcement:

The International Agency for Research on Cancer (IARC) **formally designated EMF to be a Group 2B (possible) carcinogen in humans, based on limited evidence for leukaemia in children from power line and other EMF sources**.

The IARC is regarded as the leading authority on agents raising human cancer rates in the world. The IARC – which is part of the World Health Organisation – statement took into account all previous studies to come to its conclusion. The classification was based on published scientific evidence:

"IARC has now concluded that ELF magnetic fields are possibly carcinogenic to humans, based on consistent statistical associations of high level residential magnetic fields with a doubling of risk of childhood leukaemia".[i]

The IARC had "concluded the first step in the WHO health risk assessment process by classifying ELF fields with respect to the strength of the evidence, that they could cause cancer in humans".[ii]

Our group immediately contacted the IARC.

Even though many scientists had been fighting for EMF to be classified as a 'probable' carcinogen (Group 2A) it was graded to 2B – 'possible' carcinogen. At least it had now made the list.

The IARC grading hierarchy is as follows:

- "is known to be carcinogenic to humans"   Group 1

- "is probably carcinogenic to humans" Group 2A
- "is possibly carcinogenic to humans" Group 2B
- "not classifiable as to its carcinogenicity to humans" Group 3
- "probably not carcinogenic to humans" Group 4

Tobacco smoking, tobacco smoke and asbestos are classified in Group 1.

On the WHO Fact Sheet (No. 263, October 2001) it explained that ELF fields were known to interact with tissues by inducing electric fields and currents in them, stating that this is the only established mechanism of action of these fields. This was addressing the obvious 'gross' (thermal) effects.

With this new statement the cancer risks were now finally starting to be addressed. This was a major breakthrough even though the power industry can still abide by, and most radiation bodies in the world still have guidelines that do not address cancer risks.

The electromagnetic frequency spectrum (Refer Appendix A) as we know it is divided into ionising energy and non-ionising energy:

Ionising Energy includes:

- Gamma Rays – nuclear bombs
- X-rays, CT scans, mammograms

Non-Ionising Energy includes:

- Radar
- Microwaves
- Mobile Phones and Towers
- FM Radio and Television
- AM Radio
- VDTs
- Powerlines

It has been shown that exposure to ionising radiation (even at quite low doses) could cause leukaemia. Epidemiological studies of Japanese atomic bomb survivors and *in utero* irradiation of the foetus through obstetric x-rays support this. Now the non-ionising part of the spectrum was being implicated.

In collecting and integrating biological and epidemiological evidence from all around the world Dr Cherry believed that ELF EMF is causing massive increases in cancer, cardiac, neurological and reproductive health effects. Cherry maintained that these man-made electromagnetic fields disrupt the natural production of melatonin which is the most potent natural antioxidant known to man. Produced mainly in the pineal gland melatonin – which enters every cell – was proving to be vital especially in the prevention of leukaemia and breast cancer. By disrupting melatonin our internal rhythmic processes would be disturbed leading to a cascade of events that compromises our body's defense systems which can lead to cancer.

Released mainly at night while we are sleeping, melatonin sweeps through the body eliminating the toxins that accumulate in our bodies. The ancient Egyptians and the doctors of the East revered the pineal gland referring to it as the 'third-eye' as they believed this important tiny gland, in the geometric centre of the brain, was the key to physical, mental and emotional health.

Dr Cherry contended these fields cause cancer supported by over a hundred occupational studies and over forty residential studies. He recommended the target limit chronic mean exposure level for children as 0.2mG. The desirable level in homes, schools and workplaces: 0.1mG. Cherry maintained that no level of exposure to artificial oscillating fields is safe: the safe level of exposure to 50/60 Hz fields is zero.

The vast information our group had uncovered left our group in no doubt that we had to protest against the sub-station proposal not just for ourselves but for other people we felt at risk.

The court case was drawing closer. If we were to be a part of these court proceedings we needed to engage expert witnesses. Powerlink Queensland's signed letter dated 4 September 2001 stating: "background magnetic fields in Australian homes, measured by electric utilities are typically in the range 0.5 – 5milliGauss", reinforced how important it was to fight this sub-station proposal. From our months of researching the literature in our opinion 5milliGauss was too high.

Dr Cherry had commented that the reason Doll *et al.* found a 4mG threshold, when a 2mG threshold was recommended by a US review team in the early 1990s is that all people living in these and other fields – that are significantly raising the background cancer rates – hide the effects of powerlines. Cell sites, computers and cell phones are further elevating the 'background' cancer rates.

Cherry's correspondence to our group was always concise:

> "The Australian standard is nonsense when it comes to public health because the safe level of a genotoxic carcinogen is zero and ELF fields produce cancer through reducing melatonin and through directly damaging the DNA as shown through laboratory experiments showing DNA strand breakage and chromosome aberrations".

The community co-respondents decided to present a case to the court that the court would be wise to set the limit at 2mG as the benchmark, and to demonstrate to the court there was ample evidence of increased cancer risks once exposure levels rose above 2mG for long periods of time.

Mr Alexander Doull, a Health and Safety Environment Officer employed with Australia's Commonwealth Scientific & Industrial Research Organisation (CSIRO) agreed to submit an expert report in support of our position, in the capacity of an independent consultant. Mr Doull submitted a report for our group in the interests of public health. Mr Doull did not charge the group for his work.

Corrs Chambers Westgarth retained Dr Bruce Hocking whose advice was to set a prudent avoidance at 4mG. Corrs Chambers Westgarth also engaged the services of electrical engineer, Mr Roger Lamb the electrical engineer mentioned earlier. Roger Lamb was to assess the raw data supplied by Energex.

The reports were all lodged.

The history and present stance of the experts in this court case set the stage for a compelling court case

The main experts appearing for Energex were:
- Epidemiologist, Professor Mark Elwood
- Biophysicist, Dr Andrew Wood
- Electrical Engineer, Mr Ian Shearman
- Energex EMF Expert, Mr Kevin Nuttall

Professor Elwood, the epidemiologist retained by Energex, was the present Director of the National Cancer Control Initiative, a group of cancer experts based at the Cancer Council, Victoria. The Federal Government funds the National Cancer Control Initiative to find preventative solutions to cancer. Professor Elwood was also a consultant on epidemiological issues to the Radiofrequency Exposure Standards Working Group of ARPANSA the government radiation body.

Energex also retained Andrew Wood, a biophysicist, from Swinburne University, Melbourne. Wood was part of the team that made an important discovery. Dr Wood was also involved in several Government committees and EMF matters, notably with the ARPANSA Radiation Health Committee (as Non-Ionising Radiation specialist).

Appearing for Logan City Council were:
- Specialist in Occupational Environmental Medicine, Dr Bruce Hocking
- Electrical Engineer, Mr Roger Lamb

Dr Bruce Hocking had previously been Chief Medical Officer – Corporate Industrial Relations at Telecom (Telstra) from 1977 – 1995. Hocking had been involved in what is now known as the Hocking study (1996) which "found a sixty percent increase in leukaemia in children living close to TV towers".[iii] Hocking is now a specialist in occupational environmental medicine with research interests in electromagnetic fields and other hazardous exposures in the workplace and is an Honorary Fellow with the Centre for Occupational and Environmental Health.

Roger Lamb had previously been Chief Executive Officer of the Brunswick Electricity Supply and Environmental Manager of Citipower, the Melbourne CBD electricity distributor.

Appearing for the Co-respondents was:
- Health and Safety Officer, Mr Alexander Doull.

The court case was going to be very interesting.

i   2001 www.iarc.fr/pageroot/PRELEASES/pr136a.html p.1
ii   WHO Fact Sheet 2001, p.1
iii The Parliament of the Commonwealth of Australia 2001, p.xix

Four

*I*n the lead up to the court case council's solicitors contacted us to clarify the meaning of the guidelines.

Council's solicitors were working on their case and council was stipulating fields of 2mG to Energex in their correspondence.

Energex responded to this stipulating:

> "We do not support the concept of an artificially low magnetic field strength of 2mG "safe level", which we are advised has no scientific basis. It would also appear that Logan City Council has no formal policy in this regard. The adoption of such a limit may also cause undue and unnecessary concern in the community. We are not aware of any country in the world which has adopted exposure limits differing markedly from the NHMRC (1000mG) guidelines mentioned below."

In fact, the Russians, Swedes, Swiss and the Italians had already begun the process of implementing much stricter standards.

The stage was set for a Court battle.

Case No 2604 of 2001, in November 2001 in the Planning and Environment Court, Brisbane was presided over by Judge Skoien.

COUNSEL: Lyons QC for appellant
             Gibson QC for respondent
             Donna Fisher for herself and other co-respondents

SOLICITORS: Clayton Utz for appellant
             Corrs Chambers Westgarth for respondent

DATE: 19 November 2001 – 29 November 2001

Clayton Utz was the law firm representing Energex. Barrister, Peter Lyons, was acting as QC for Energex.

Corrs Chambers Westgarth was the law firm representing Logan City Council and had employed barrister, Graham Gibson, in the capacity of QC.

With no knowledge of the law or how the court case would run, I represented the co-respondents in the daunting courtroom experience. Clayton Utz and Corrs Chambers Westgarth had barristers, solicitors, junior solicitors and clerks assisting them. Jenny Cadwallader assisted me. Cheryl, a schoolteacher and one of the team, was most disappointed she could not attend.

DAY ONE

Court commenced at 10am. Silence in Court.

Case begins and as Energex was the appellant they opened the case.

It was acknowledged that Logan City in South East Queensland had grown enormously and quickly in the last ten years. The need for a sub-station was a necessity. The new Loganholme Hyperdome Shopping Centre, which had been marketed as the largest shopping centre in the southern hemisphere on one level, was across the highway from where we lived. A new hospital had also been constructed three kilometres away.

In the afternoon session it was determined that the judge and Peter Lyons and Graham Gibson and myself would visit the proposed site. We looked at other possible sub-station sites that were further away from residential houses. Attention was brought to an older sub-station that was in an industrial estate far away from any residential houses.

DAY TWO

This day was about why Energex chose the proposed site as opposed to other sites. Peter Lyons, Graham Gibson and I cross-examined Energex staff in their choice of the proposed site. The epicentre of the demand for electricity turned out to be in the vicinity of the Logan Hyperdome Shopping Centre. There was a vacant block of land at this location yet it was an extremely valuable block of land.

DAY THREE

This was the day when the Electrical Engineer for Energex, Ian Shearman, was to appear.

Peter Lyons cross-examined first, followed by Graham Gibson and then myself.

During my cross examination Ian Shearman confirmed that the

Soviet Government had introduced the first standards addressing the biological effects and incorporated this more cautious approach for limiting such EMF exposure as early as the late 1950s. Shearman also confirmed the 1.5mG Russian standard.

During cross-examination the judge became aware of the differences between the 'gross' (thermal) effects and the 'subtle' (biological) effects to which he directed questions to Shearman as well.

Point 23 in Professor Elwood's expert report stated:

> "These guidelines represent the acceptable levels of exposure for the general public to electric and magnetic fields of the type experienced here, and are based on an understanding of the levels of exposure which can cause health effects, plus a substantial safety margin to ensure that the guideline levels are well below the levels which can produce effects on health. The relevant guideline set by the NHMRC is 1000mG."

I now believed that the references to the 'health effects' were understood more clearly.

On asking Shearman if his projected figures had taken into account the addition of a third sub-station in the future it appeared that Mr Shearman was not aware of a possible future third transformer. This had been an anomaly Cheryl had found in a report from 'discovery' which was when we were able to view the other party's documents before the court proceedings.

After Shearman left the stand, Energex Barrister Peter Lyons requested to stand down the matter. We waited for many hours as there were serious discussions taking place between the Energex and Corrs Chambers Westgarth barristers and solicitors. We were then advised we could leave as settlement terms were still being negotiated. It was my understanding that there was a proposal to settle the matter by agreeing that where reasonably possible, the sub-station and powerlines would not exceed an 'average' level of 4mG at the residential property boundaries.

Late into the night the solicitors were hard at work to come to a settlement. Roger Lamb, representing Logan City Council was advising Council on field strengths and emissions. Energex tabled their calculating systems during this period and Roger Lamb was accumulating very valuable data which had never been presented outside of the power companies.

It became apparent to our group that the 'time averaging' method used by Energex served only to dilute the periods of more intense exposures. Even though an individual may be exposed to a 26mG field for some hours and 0mG for other hours, it will be 'averaged' over a 24-hour period, diluting it down. The figures were then 'averaged' again over 365 days and as long as the 'average' is below 4mG, all is well. We saw it as a method to allow for increased exposures as 'averages' were usually taken only over a 24 hour period.

A 24 hour 'average' was still being used, but instead of the addition of the 365 day 'average', it was my understanding that Roger Lamb, council, Graham Gibson and Energex were working on bringing that 'average' closer to a truer measurement.

DAY FOUR

Judge Skoien commented on the lack of legal representation in the courtroom. The chief solicitors were absent as settlement talks were still being held throughout the day and late into the night. It was time for Professor Elwood to take the stand even though the settlement that was being worked on was unprecedented. Elwood had to take the stand and was cross-examined first by Peter Lyons for Energex.

Graham Gibson, in his cross-examination of Professor Elwood was brilliant. On closing his cross-examination of Professor Elwood, Graham Gibson asked:

> **"Incidentally, I take it in giving your evidence, Professor; you don't do so in your capacity as director of the National Cancer Control Initiative?"**
>
> **Elwood's reply:** "No".
>
> **Gibson: "So as they say in the disclaimers the opinions are yours not those of that organisation?"**
>
> **Elwood:** "That's true".

It was my turn to cross-examine Professor Elwood.

As my expert believed the benchmark should be 2mG, I had to ask one of the most important questions which was if there was any statistical evidence associated with ELF EMF and childhood cancer between exposures of 2mG and 4mG.

On Jenny bringing attention to me that I did not include the very important word 'statistical' in my original question I had to further:

> **"Professor Elwood is there any statistical evidence associated with ELF EMFs and childhood cancer between exposures of 2mG and 4mG?" You said "Yes. Is that correct?"**
>
> **Elwood replied:** "That's right there is some evidence but there is not consistent evidence which supports causality".
>
> **"According to your opinion?"**
>
> **Elwood replied:** "My opinion and others".

I have since noticed that the word 'statistical' in the second question was not typed into the transcript.

DAY FIVE

Andrew Wood, the biophysicist appearing for Energex was cross-examined by Peter Lyons and Graham Gibson. Once again Graham Gibson's skills were admirable. I asked only three questions of Dr Wood:

> **Is there any evidence that the suppression of the functioning of the pineal gland leads to increased occurrence of tumours of the breast in animals or humans?**
>
> **Wood's reply:** This was a theory that was in vogue a few years ago, and certainly there was some evidence to show that high levels of melatonin act as a free radical scavenger and the assumption was that if you remove free radicals the possibility of tumours developing would be less, but it turned out that the amount of melatonin that you need in order to produce this free radical scavenging is so large that it wouldn't be a mechanism that would be normally operating.
>
> **Is there any evidence that electromagnetic fields suppress the functioning of the pineal gland?**
>
> **Wood's reply:** Well, yes, some of our own work has sort of, shown that, but as I said nobody else has been able to get a similar result to us. So we aren't – whenever one produces scientific study in which you find a positive outcome you still leave open the possibility that that could be due to statistical chance, and the fact that nobody else seems to have got a similar result to us would make us believe that, perhaps, our results were due to statistical variation rather than the real effect.

Our research had revealed that ELF EMF fields operated at 50 Hertz and we had come across information that it had been found that one of the most important processes of our bodies – calcium ions – has been shown to operate around the same frequency. Even though this was shown in a mathematical model and concepts in mathematics are often way ahead of science, while we had the chance to ask a scientist who had been party to this discovery I further asked:

Did you participate in research which discovered a fundamental calcium ion resonance at 50.1 Hertz or in that vicinity?

Wood's reply: Yes, the theoretical study that we did with Colin Thompson showed that you could get – in theory anyway, you could get reasonable phenomena at a number of frequencies, but as I said previously, the conditions under which that mechanism would operate are not the conditions that exist inside the human body. So it was a mathematical – it was published because of its mathematical interest rather than that it had direct relevance to human physiology, and I make that point in here.

Day Five was over.

In regard to the once controversial association with tobacco smoking and cancer, and the controversial association between asbestos and cancer, the cross-examinations by Graham Gibson put this health issue into context.

The settlement was still being worked on over the weekend.

On Sunday afternoon I received a call at home from a solicitor at Clayton Utz, stating that Energex and council had signed off on a settlement. The solicitor asked if the co-respondents still wanted to proceed with the case.

The settlement was an incredulous achievement in itself. Even though our small group was disappointed that the sub-station was still to be constructed so close to our homes it was an extraordinary advance – 4mG instead of 1000mG was to be used as a guideline for the design and construction.

The 'averaging' method used by Energex to dilute exposures was addressed. 'Averaging' which is often criticized is usually done over a 24 hour period. Instead of the measurements being 'averaged' over 24 hours and then again 'averaged' over 365 days of the year, they were now 'averaged' over 24 hours and only two months of the year. The months of June and December were selected. Even though our group still felt it was still a diluted measurement it was a major advance. This was a major concession.

Most importantly, the council had the right to request verified readings so they could monitor the situation. We were advised that this was the only case in the world where a sub-station had limits imposed on it and the fields within the community also limited.

In short, the sub-station was to go ahead on the proposed block of land with strict stipulations:

> The fields emanating from the sub-station were not allowed to go over 4mG and the fields in six different locations in the community were also to be kept at 4mG, where reasonably practical.

> Limits were placed on the ultimate capacity of the sub-station site. Only two transformers were allowed and their capacity limited.

> Even though the EMF was to be limited at the sub-station it would be significantly higher where certain cables entered or left the sub-station and where the associated feeders pass overhead though the surrounding community. This was addressed and certain feeders and powerlines were to be under-grounded with strict stipulations on their configuration and covering.

The conditions Energex must adhere to are comprehensive and meticulous.

Even though council and Energex had signed off on a settlement, our group decided to continue on. It was now Energex versus the co-respondents and the case continued for two more days. Six weeks later, judgment was handed down in January 2002. The settlement was made an Order of the Court. It was a world first as said by Doull ... "a very important decision, a **world first**".

SOME THOUGHTS . . .

UP CLOSE & PERSONAL

When our group fought the sub-station proposal we had no idea that we would be thrown into a court case of such magnitude. Writing a simple letter of protest which culminated in experiencing the dreaded legal system was indeed a life-changing experience.

When our group attended the first meeting with Energex and council at council chambers Ted Fensom spoke about environmental concerns and Jim Kerr spoke about community aspects. After I spoke about my reasons for objecting to the sub-station I stated loud and clear to Energex: "I WON'T BACK DOWN". And I didn't.

*At the state level, on visiting the Labor politician Tom Barton about relocating the sub-station **Tom stated that I should stay in the kitchen and not bother myself about things like this**. I believed Tom Barton thought I was the "Not In My Back Yard" type implying I did not care if the sub-station was close to others.*

Cr Pam Parker, tall with long flowing blonde hair, very-well dressed and always available made us feel she would protect us under any fearful circumstance. With her compassionate and no-nonsense attitude Pam, I felt, was a successful blend of feminine and masculine principles. (Present day September 2007 Pam came over to my house to ask me if I would be one of her six campaign women as she had decided to run for Mayor. Pam won and is now Mayor of Logan City).

Some months before the court case Cr Pam Parker invited our group for a meeting at council chambers. Jenny and Greg, Cheryl and Jim, Cameron and myself, David Turner and a couple of other team members attended. Cr Pam Parker was there along with Leanne Bowman from Corrs Westgarth Chambers. Leanne Bowman advised us that we (I believed this to be council and the co-respondents) had a 20% chance of winning the case and put forth the idea that maybe we should think more realistically about the situation. The planning case was weak. (The power companies can put sub-stations and powerlines anywhere they like....)

Cheryl Kerr angrily demanded that council sack their lawyers and engage new ones.

We were feisty but disappointed. We had no funds to fight this proposal and all other avenues had been exhausted. Was this the end of our fight?

It was not long after this that Cr Pam Parker advised me about the telecommunications conference where Mr Bangay from ARPANSA spoke which gave us the important Dr Cherry lead. This put our group on a whole new path and more experts in this field who answered my many questions.

On being advised on the qualifications of electrical engineer, Roger Lamb I rang him many times and often into the late of night. Roger, a mine-field of information was very patient and very understanding of our plight.

It was Roger who advised me about the misunderstanding of the guidelines. When Cheryl and I fully comprehended what this meant and the importance of it, it was then that we as a group got very busy.

Cheryl and I wrote to Premier Peter Beattie, every member of the Energex board personally and to Corrs Chambers and Westgarth. In our letter we directed them to the how the present guidelines did not address the cancer risk and we stated firmly:

> *"There was 'something in the food', 'there was something in the water', 'there was something in the cigarettes' and now there is 'something in the air'".*

Energex replied acknowledging the 'slight risk of leukaemia'.

Leanne Bowman from Corrs Chambers Westgarth contacted me and asked for clarification of the guidelines again and suddenly the outlook changed. Council's solicitors went into overdrive. The fight was on!

All the way through Sandy Doull said although he would help us with information as an independent consultant he was unable put in an 'expert witness report'. He currently worked for the CSIRO. I believed it may put his job at risk, though I never did ask.

As I had booked a holiday much earlier I went overseas for two weeks in early October with not long to go before the court case. I left it with Cheryl to find an expert witness out of nowhere. Six weeks before the court case and we still did not have an expert witness.

On my return Cheryl announced that she had handed into the court an 'expert witness report' from the originally reluctant Sandy Doull. On asking her how she convinced him she simply stated: "I told him we were desperate". Sandy Doull prepared the report within 36 hours to meet the deadline. An amazing feat!! This court case was going to be very interesting.

I was nervous but never faltered in my belief that I had to fight to the end. I was concerned though as I was not of quick mind and one to counter back. Even though I was in my early forties I hated confrontation. I was the type who stood in the shower a few nights later stating what I should have said at the time.

We were told that Peter Lyons – barrister for Energex – had been a Jesuit priest in training to some degree. I wondered why some-one with this background would represent a power company. Strange bedfellows!!

I thought – by the time I'm finished with him he will have wished he was on council's side.

It was alleged that Professor Ellwood who was an expert witness for Energex was being paid by the Federal Government to find preventative solutions to cancer for Australians. It was also alleged that he was also being paid by the power companies. Was he on two payrolls? This brought the term 'moonlighting' to a new level. Sleeping with the enemy!!!! The IARC statement had been announced only a few months earlier but he was substituting his own judgment over the highest cancer authority in the world. Ellwood has been a consultant to the IARC. ELF EMF only got to be classed as a Group 2B carcinogen – apparently the fights across the room from scientists were enormous at the time. I wonder, does he sleep?   When the Wertheimer Leeper study had been repeated and confirmed the electrical industry in Australia in the 1980s looked for a cancer specialist who would befriend them. It is said that they found him.

Ellwood popped up in court cases for the telecommunications companies as well as the power companies. There were only a very small handful of men around the world who represented the power companies but they were strategically placed on certain organisations. Both Ellwood and Wood had positions within our radiation board.

Graham Gibson – barrister for Council – had the demeanour of a cool operator.

Dr Bruce Hocking appearing for Council had been Chief Medical Officer for Telecom (Telstra) for eighteen years. Hocking conducted a study to investigate any link between serious disease and communication towers. Hocking now specialised in occupational environmental medicine with a special interest in these silent fields.

Sandy Doull and I were a team. He had so much knowledge but was helping a small group who were so far out of their depth.

* *

The Court Case

Day One

I decided that I needed to act and dress like an advocate so I dressed in corporate black – top, skirt, jacket, stocking, shoes – with a briefcase at my side. From early on I had decided that I had to act like those I was joining ranks with for a while...sort of fake it until you make it!

When Clayton Utz needed to give me some documents in a hurry before the court case I was having lunch at the very old-school Tattersall's Club. I asked them to deliver the documents to me there. I was not some underclass scrubber!!

In the morning session they really just ignored me. The judge and the two barristers were in conversation. I wondered if it was because most co-respondents are seen as vexatious.

Anyway it was decided that they would visit the area where we lived. I asked if I could come along and they all just looked at me in surprise. I stated that I needed a lift home anyway as I had been dropped off. So we all hopped in the car.

*Peter Lyons was driving, Judge Skoien in the front passenger seat, Graham Gibson and myself in the back. So there I was in the car and well maybe I chatted a little too much but I needed to tell the judge that I stuttered slightly and that if I looked like I could not pronounce a word – especially for example 'epidemiology' it was because I stuttered on my d's not because of my intellect or inability to spell. I had to then further explain how from a young age I stuttered on every letter but it was now only by d's and my b's. (I had licked 24 letters, 2 stubborn ones to go). **And I thought I could do this, what was I thinking?***

We drove around the area and I showed them where a sub-station was in an industrial estate – far away from houses.

After the tour they dropped me home and I will always remember stating: "See you tomorrow". It was then that I remembered my father's words over the years: "Donna you have more front than Myer".

Came home to a house full of hungry children and a husband that does not cook – they didn't really understand the day.

Day Two

I dressed again like the enemy.

This was the day about why they chose the site and Lyons, Gibson and I cross-examined. The epicentre of the demand turned out to be in the vicinity of the huge newer shopping centre across the road. The block of land there was extremely valuable. The block of land in our street was much cheaper. It always comes back to the dollar!!

Day Three

I knew Mr Shearman being an electrical engineer would not expect questions on the health issue but would know them. Electricians are not educated in the risks associated with these fields. Electrical engineers are though.

So I wore a pink jacket that day knowing that body language and appearance can make a difference. I actually talked to him before court started acting quite innocent.

When he was on the stand my questions were of intent. I actually argued with the judge during this as Peter Lyons was arguing that I was crossing into epidemiology and it was not appropriate. I think in the end it was stated that Mr Shearman was not an epidemiologist.

The judge had also told me that my sentences were so long it was as though I was trying to tell a story. Still I got the answers to my questions.

When I asked if his figures had incorporated a third transformer/sub-station in the future he looked totally bewildered!!

When the judge asked how I had come across this information I stated it had been found through the "discovery" process in a report on page 5. Even though Jenny and I had gone into Clayton Utz's office and photocopied documents, Cheryl examined the documents most carefully picking up this anomaly and setting the questions for Shearman.

After Shearman's testimony, Peter Lyons asked for the case to be shut down. The lawyers and barristers were in deep discussion. Energex obviously did not want Ellwood and Wood to take the stand while it was obvious they were discussing going from 1000mG to 4mG.

After quite a while Roger Lamb and Graham Gibson were standing beside Jenny and me. Roger stated that a 4mG was being proposed. I remember blurting out: "What about the children, it is 2mG"? Later I looked Graham Gibson in the eye and stated: "I am in this until council get what they want and until I get what I want". Graham Gibson did warn not to 'grandstand' though.

Discussions were going well into the night which Graham Gibson also advised the judge of one day.

Day Four

Where was everyone? The legal teams were sparse as they were concentrating on settlement terms. Even the judge commented.

This day esteemed Professor Ellwood hit the stand. He had to stand by his report. When Ellwood walked into the courtroom and headed straight towards Peter Lyons the barrister and asked: "How switched on is the judge to all this?" I was shocked. Jenny also heard it. I felt sick, extremely nervous and wanted to crawl out of the room. What was I doing here against the big boys?

Ellwood's voice was so monotone as though he had said these words over and over throughout the years. He was skilled. Peter Lyons cross-examined for such a long time.

Graham Gibson in his cross-examination was great giving him a good whiplashing. I loved his closing questions!!

Well it was my turn to cross-examine and I had so many questions I was a wreck. He was so skilled and I was trying to keep myself together. After a few questions and fumbling at them the judge motioned for a break when I tried to compose myself.

I came in and asked one question (after lots of coaching from Jenny in the break):

"Professor Elwood is there any statistical evidence associated with ELF EMFs and childhood cancer between exposures of 2mG and 4mG?"

You said, "Yes. Is that correct?"

Elwood replied: *"That's right there is some evidence but there is not consistent evidence which supports causality".*

"According to your opinion?"

Elwood replied: *"My opinion and others".*

My unspoken thoughts at the time: Anyway, it is not necessary to identify a biological mechanism for classifying a causal effect (Hill 1965). Dr Hocking will sort that out!!! You are an epidemiologist and epidemiology does not show causality.

Day Five

As with the Ellwood cross-examination Peter Lyons took what seemed hours to cross-examine Wood.

Graham Gibson gave him a good whiplashing as well. Gibson really caught onto the subject very quickly. I liked immensely his no-nonsense attitude. Gibson asked Wood a question which everyone was surprised to hear his answer. Can't remember it though even though Roger Lamb bought it to my attention and Sandy Doull may know also.

It was my turn to cross-examine.

Now during the court process the judge had given me a tip. He told me in front of the court room that if you cross-examine your witness for too long it weakens your case. I thought that if this was the case Peter Lyons had been doing that all along. So I kept my questions brief. I only asked three questions of Wood.

Day Five questioning was over and I clearly remember Peter Lyons walking up to me and asking me **"Do you think the people of Australia will ever realise what you have done for them?"** *I think I replied: "No, not really". I was quite taken aback. He also asked me if I had an idea of what the case would be like. I commented that it was like a marriage, you didn't really know what it was like until you were in it and no one could describe how it really is. I wondered why I used that analogy. I knew he would wish he was on our side!*

Settlement talks were being held all over the weekend. I was not privy to these. On Sunday afternoon John from Clayton Utz rang to inform me that a settlement had been signed off between Energex and council. **I thought so. Dr Hocking does not have to take the stand**. *He enquired as to whether we would still go on. As Cheryl, Jenny and I were so adamantly opposed to the sub-station being still so close to our houses we decided to fight on.*

Ian Wright, head partner from Corrs Chambers Westgarth came to my house and congratulated me.

Sandy Doull telephoned to confirm his need to testify. I asked him if we could get into the science of it – the pineal gland and melatonin, and the 50 Hertz calcium ion resonance. Sandy Doull's advice was to hold back stating: "not to bite the whole cherry". He stated that what we had achieved had been amazing, a world first and that was enough for now. As we all thought he would be appearing earlier in the case he could not make it up to Queensland so he gave me his telephone number at home as the court would have to call him for cross-examination.

Day Six

Council were now not involved. Leanne Bowman was the only one present from Corrs Chambers Westgarth now and Leanne sat in the courtroom along the front with Lyons and myself but did not partake in any proceedings.

Peter Lyons cross-examined Peter Priddell the planning expert as did I. Cheryl attended this day as she was to be cross-examined herself. She also provided the questions for Priddell. I knew my EMF but I was not interested in the planning argument. It was all too much information for me when I was struggling to keep myself together throughout this ordeal. I cross-examined him briefly with my main argument being that he had based all of his work on assuming the guidelines were for biological effects which they were not. The judge steered me away from this though.

Next was Kevin Nuttall the EMF expert at Energex. I really didn't ask him many questions as I had been advised not to ask a question that you don't know what the answer is going to be. Anyway I had lost a whole night sleep on Wednesday night – after Day Three – and was only getting about 3 hours a night. I definitely am an 8 hour girl!! Peter Lyons later commented to me that I went soft on Nuttall.

Next was the cross-examination of our expert Sandy Doull. On my way in the car that morning John from Clayton Utz had rang me on my mobile and said he needed to send Sandy Doull some paperwork. Just before Sandy was to be phoned by the court for his cross-examination they faxed Sandy lots of paper work which he had to fudge through. I cross-examined with my brief questions keeping in mind the judge's previous comments about not cross-examining your own witness for too long. It was off-putting asking questions over the phone anyway. Peter Lyons on his turn was really frustrating. Sandy with his raspy voice kept repeating that examination of all the studies had already been done for the IARC to come to its conclusion. He sounded exasperated. The judge commented in his judgment that Sandy had overstated his case. I could see why!! Peter Lyons was dragging it all out in his usual style. I felt like throwing a bucket of water over him myself.

*Near the end of the day the judge said that summation would be tomorrow. I stated that I thought I had a week. He stated: "No". The judge then asked me how I thought this and wanted to know if someone involved in the court case had told me. I advised him that neither Energex nor council representatives had advised me of this. I had received free legal advice in the build-up to the court case and this is what I was advised. **So much for free advice – you only get what you pay for**. The fact being that I did not know what to expect each day. I just kept turning up!!*

I rushed home to prepare for summation. Well everything went wrong. I came home to a testy family who were fed-up with an absent mother and take-away meals. My daughter was also in the middle of important school exams. My computer was playing up.

Looking back I cannot remember whether the judge granted a full day off or if I turned up to court on the next day – Tuesday – at 10am and I told the judge I was not ready. Either way I remember that the judge asked Peter Lyons if Wednesday was okay for him. Lyons agreed.

I went home and collapsed on the bed for a few hours then the children came home and life as always was full on. When Cheryl got home from work I asked her to type up the planning case and I was doing the EMF. Half way into the night my printer wouldn't work.

After a few hours sleep I tried again, got the printer working for a while but needed more copies of the summation. I rang Greg and he went to a photo-copying store. He seemed to take such a long time. I felt as though I was in a time-warp. He picked me up and we were running late. He seemed to drive so slowly. He was safe though and this is what I needed. Calm amongst the storm. It was ten o'clock and we still were not in the city. When we arrived I rushed up the stairs and entered the court room at 10.11am. Leanne Bowman looked really nice that day and I remember complimenting her. Why I do not know. Anyway there were more people from Energex here today. **Were they really that interested in what I had to say?**

The judge came into the room now I had arrived. I told him everything had gone wrong and apologised. I also did not expect anymore leniency and felt disrespectful.

Well I stood up and went blank for a few moments. Then I spoke. I can't remember a lot but it just poured out of my mouth. I remember arguing with the judge to cause him to say: "Mrs Fisher I am only hotly debating with you". There I was with my hands on my hips aggressively arguing about the diluted measurements.

The time weighted average system is criticized as it is over a 24 hour period. These guys then diluted the measurements even more by diluting them again over a 365 day period. I felt they were not only rewriting science, it was maths as well!

The judge commented that wasn't it now improved as it was only now over two months of the year instead of 365 days. He also stated that the months of June and December were picked – the two months of highest energy consumption. I told him that it was still 4.5mG in the centre of our narrow road. (My children's bedrooms were at the front of the house which was very close to the road).

(In a late night phone call to Roger Lamb after the settlement he advised me that the measurement was still 4.5mG in the centre of the road.)

I also argued that as it is officially quoted that these fields affect a few children in every 100,000, if you add up all the children in the world that is a lot of children.

Then it was over. I looked at the clock and wondered how the time went so fast. I had been talking for quite some time. The experience was so surreal. When I first spoke I felt as though someone else had entered my body and was doing the talking. I felt like I was floating. They did not seem like my words. I will never forget the odd feeling I felt that morning, it is hard to explain. Might have to keep this to myself though!!!

The court went for a break.

I was still holding myself together somehow when one of the Energex men came over to me to ask me how I was. What do you do when you are just holding it together and someone asks you how you are? That was when I started crying. I escaped into the ladies room. There I sat crying and on my own as Jenny was not with me this day. I was still crying when we had to return to the court room. Actually I was sobbing uncontrollably. The pressure of the build-up, trying to find someone to help us, the need for an expert and having no funds was finally taking its toll. It had been a hard fight and I was now totally exhausted. A few hours each night and a total lack of sleep on one night had done me in.

So there I was with Peter Lyons doing his summation and sobbing the whole way through. Leanne Bowman handed me her handkerchief. I could not stop crying so I walked towards the exit door. The judge commented that he would have to stop the case if I left the room so I returned to my seat. I was so disappointed with myself.

After Peter Lyon's summation I was allowed comment on his summation. This I did not know. I thought in my haze that Lyons had slighted my expert so I mentioned this yet the judge confirmed that Sandy Doull had been a competent witness.

The judge frustratingly asked Lyons and me if we could explain what the problem with these fields was. He was exasperated. I knew it in my head but I could not get the words out. Sandy Doull had advised me to leave the science alone. He had stated: "You have achieved enough Donna, it is unprecedented". So I did. I was finding it hard to string a sentence together anyway.

It was over.

The judge's last words: "Mrs Fisher, go home and get some sleep". What an inappropriate remark! Paternalism?

* *

Early January 2002, six weeks later the judge's assistant rang me to advise when judgment was being handed down. I stated I was on Hamilton Island for the month and to apologise to the judge as I could not attend. Cheryl, Jim, Jenny and Greg attended though.

Cheryl rang with the bad news that the sub-station was to still go ahead. On staying on the court case as Energex v Co-respondents in those last two days we were still fighting against the location of the sub-station. Some felt it was a LOSS. I though felt it was a WIN. A win for the people so it could be quoted far and wide that 4mG not 1000mG was to be used as a guideline in the planning of the sub-station. This could enable others to achieve the same to protect them. Sandy Doull and Roger Lamb were elated. Dr Hocking was also pleased. Even though it seemed a small step for us, it was huge in the EMF world. It was a WORLD FIRST. 'Microwave News' in New York even wrote an article on the outcome.

We all moved house after that. The house next door to the sub-station which Energex in the courtroom referred to as the 'derelict' house where no-one would live still has people living in it.

As I look back now many years later I am concerned about the corona ion effect theory of Professor Henshaw. We did not pay much attention to this at the time but if he is correct and he looks like he may be the corona ions from the sub-station would affect the nearby residents as well. The magnetic fields are addressed but not the corona ion effect.

What made me persist so much to be called 'tenacious' by Pam Parker and her want me along on her campaign in later years?

I do not know. I believe it may have been the fact that Cheryl, Jenny and I acted as such a strong force together. Even though I was four and twelve years their junior it was three women thinking of their own families and other families together that forged a bond that could not be broken. We were supported by each other's strengths and refused to give in to our weaknesses. For example, my life-long stutter and my life-long distaste for confrontation did not stop me from standing up in court against learned men. Jenny who also questioned her ability to cross-examine witnesses gave me support throughout the court case each day at my side. Cheryl with her excellent command of the English language and her sharp mind would have been a far superior cross-examiner but being a school teacher she could not attend. Cheryl wrote the questions for Shearman and Priddle. None of us even talked about it much to other people afterwards. We just thought that this is what human beings are supposed to do, that it wasn't anything extraordinary.

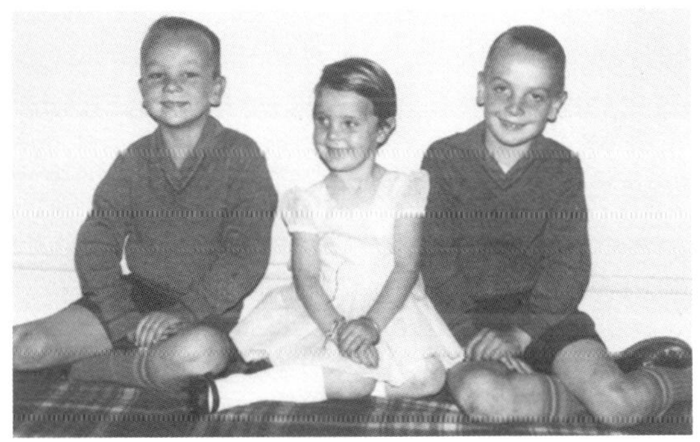

Donna at 4 years old with her brothers

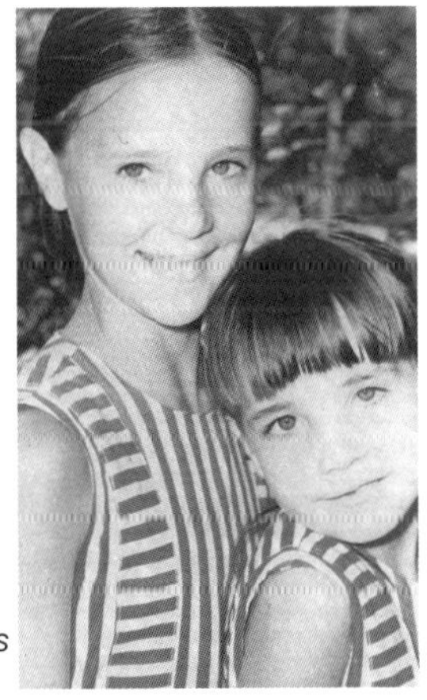

Donna at 12 years old with her younger sister. Donna's protective nature was noticed from an early age.

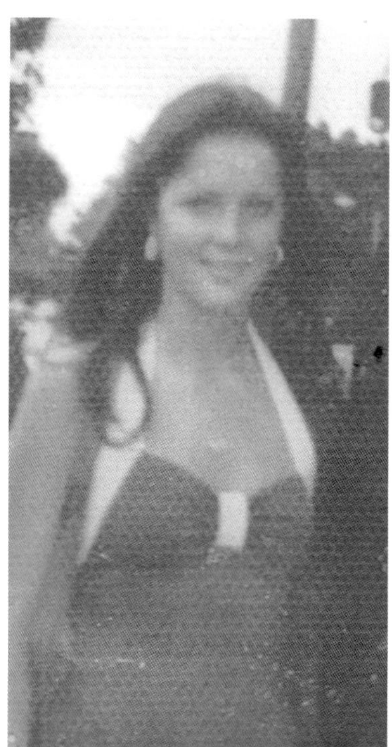

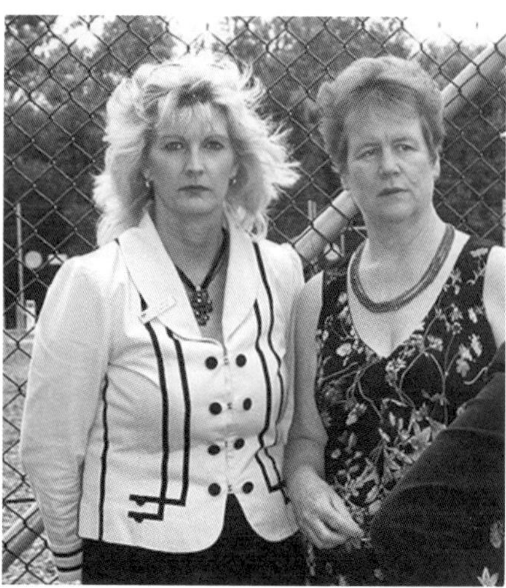

Mayor Pam Parker and Cheryl Kerr outside the sub-station in Sewell Road.

A young and carefree Donna in her teenage years but filled with discovery of the world.

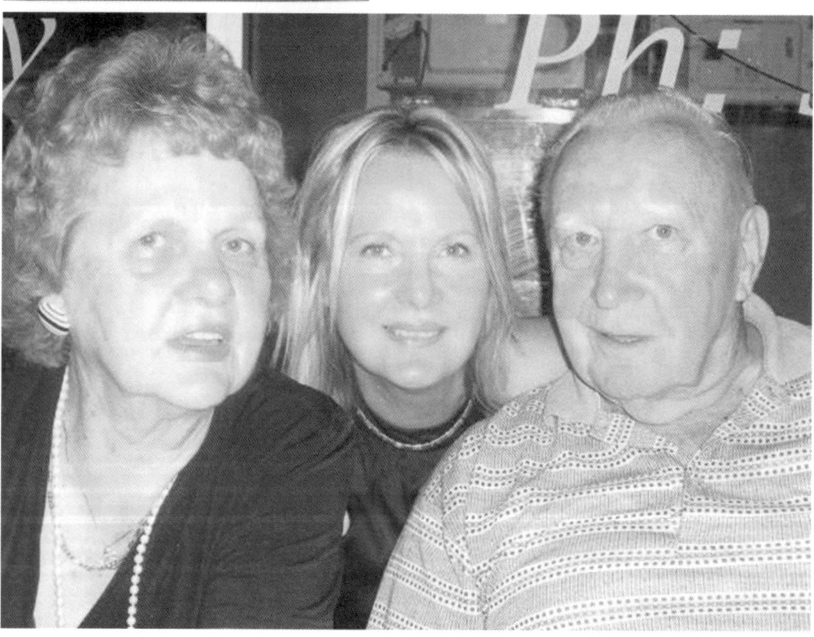

Donna with her parents – really important pillars in her life.

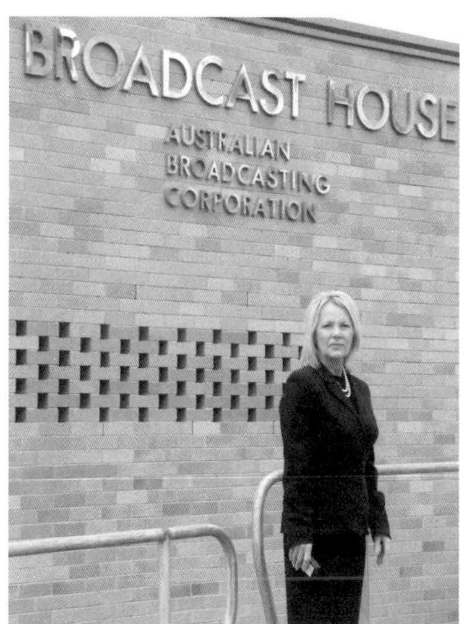
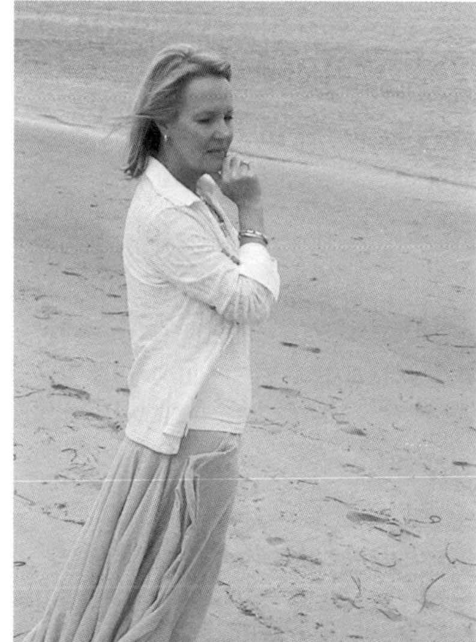

At the ABC studio. Measuring for "dirty" electricity can be quite a simple process!

Top right:
Never one to seek attention, Donna walking along her favourite beach wondering how much resistance on this issue she would encounter.

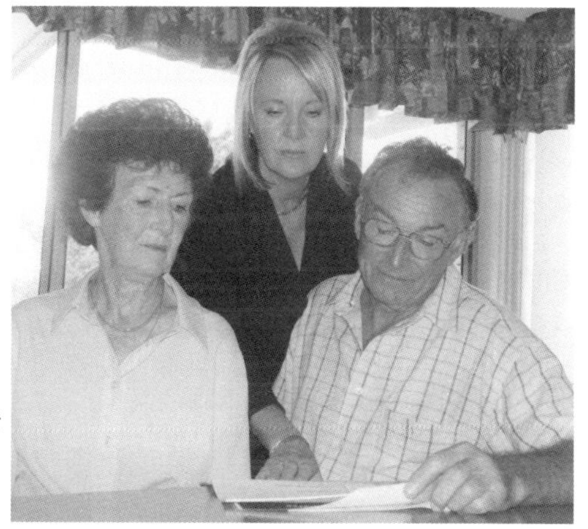

Donna with neighbours Jenny and Greg Cadwallader perusing information from overseas scientists which played a significant role in defining the problem and offering solutions.

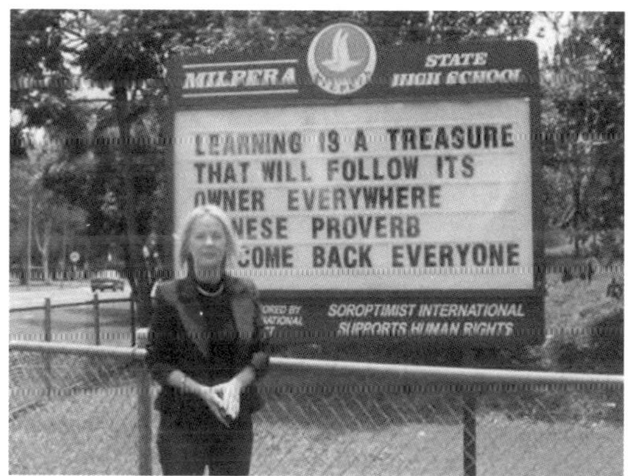

On site at Milpera State High School – seeking to help through critical information.

Five

$\mathcal{E}$arlier it was reported on how industry sceptics appeared to disregard the views of Neil Cherry implying perhaps that he was some kind of fringe group guru. Character assassination no less, the machine was working.

The injustice of such an interpretation was exposed five weeks after our court case, on 1 January 2002, when Dr Cherry was awarded the Royal Honour of Officer of New Zealand Order of Merit (O.N.Z.M.) for his services to Science, Education and Community. An elected Regional Councillor on Environmental, Canterbury this recognition included reference to his research and teaching work on environmental epidemiology and the health effects of electromagnetic radiation.

Meanwhile the other expert, electrical engineer Roger Lamb who appeared for Logan City Council, prepared a report on our court case, stating it provided an important precedent and a model for the resolution of similar situations in the future. His report stated: "the data presented clearly shows that under day-to-day operating conditions, as identified, it is possible for individuals in homes or businesses throughout Australia that are adjacent to overhead feeders and distribution transformers, to be subjected to long-term exposure of fields in excess of 4mG".[i]

A proposal to construct a new library next door to a sub-station was stopped by Logan City Council. Cr Pam Parker was still fighting to protect local citizens by bringing attention to another property where the powerlines in the backyard were within 7 metres from a bedroom. The young girl who grew up in this room commenced her menstrual cycle at an exceptionally early age. Recently it was discovered that this lady's young son, now seven years of age, has been riddled with tumours from very early in his life. He had slept in this same room most nights. Now better informed on magnetic field measurements, Pam Parker enquired about the field emissions when hearing that the fields from these powerlines were being upgraded by Energex.

On measuring magnetic fields with equipment that measures these fields (gaussmeter) in two different homes extremely close to powerlines the following results presented: The first household, in a lower socio-economic suburb had powerlines running within 7 metres of the bedrooms. Fields of 4.4mG were measured in the bedroom, where two girls under four years of age were sleeping. This is a concern. The other household, in an affluent suburb, had powerlines within 7 metres of their home. I recorded in the living room and the two teenage bedrooms fields of 7.8mG and 8mG. Once again, this is a major concern.

A more recent Japanese study found high magnetic fields in the bedroom (exposed to 4mG or more) could increase the risk of childhood leukaemia by up to nearly five times. Week long measurements were taken as well as spot measurements.

(Refer Kabuto, M. *et al*. International Journal of Cancer, February 22 2006).

In 2002 not far from our area, the Benson family in the Gold Coast hinterland with two small children and three teenagers refused to allow Powerlink access to their property as Powerlink intended to construct major powerlines within 50 metres. Powerlink instigated legal proceedings. In January 2003, Professor Mark Elwood and Dr Andrew Wood submitted expert reports on behalf of Powerlink – Supreme Court of Queensland S7414/02.

A more damning report from the Department of Health Services, California was released after our court case. In August 2002, the Californian Department of Health Services (DHS) presented its 8 year $7million EMF Program Risk Assessment Report Summary. The conclusions of the scientists were, in part, that all three were *"inclined to believe that EMFs can cause some degree of increased risk of childhood leukaemia, adult brain cancer, Lou Gehrig's Disease, and miscarriage".*

(*Executive Summary of the California EMF Risk Evaluation For Policymakers And the Public*, The California Department of Health Services, June 2002).

It was not only the Benson family who understood the importance of the California Department of Health Services (CDHS) report, lawyers for the electrical industry also took note. Watson and Renner, an influential law firm based in Washington, USA and Legal Counsel to the UHSG (Utilities Health Sciences Group) distributed advice to

UHSG members 14 June 2002 that:

> It is possible to argue that the CDHS conclusion does not say explicitly that there is an established cause and effect relationship between EMF and any disease. **We believe, however, that the CDHS conclusion is sufficiently close to causation that a global statement that none of the science reviews concludes there is a causal relationship would be legally inadvisable**.

Many of the electrical utilities throughout the world are members of the UHSG (including the ESAA – Australia).

Margaret and Geoff Benson handed me this document which was obtained when they were granted 'discovery' of Powerlink's records. They did this so others could benefit.

The Need for Clarification of the Guidelines

The assumption that 1000mG exposures are safe, therefore there is no possible cancer risk occurs quite frequently. In 2002 at the Royal Women's Hospital in Melbourne, Victoria, magnetic fields of above 250mG were found in the day-care crèche for staff where sixteen children aged from ten months to four years spent their day. This room was located directly above the hospital's electricity sub-station. When the current guidelines were understood more clearly the crèche was re-located.

The statement often used is: "at no point did the measured ELF magnetic fields exceed the General Public Limits of the NHMRC guidelines". Compliance to the current guidelines does not relate to cancer risk. The current guidelines in Australia (and most other countries) are 1000mG and do not address the leukaemia, brain tumour or breast cancer risk.

In May 2006, the RMIT University in Victoria took the unprecedented step of vacating the two top floors of Building 108 at its Bourke Street campus where a number of senior staff worked. Five staff members in April and May 2006 were found to have brain tumours, as well as two others in 1999 and 2001.

Professor Mark Elwood, head of the National Cancer Control Initiative at the Cancer Council Victoria, stated he thought that coincidence was *"the most likely explanation"* in regard to the RMIT University case.[ii]

In also referring to the RMIT University case, John Loy, CEO of the Australian Radiation Protection & Nuclear Safety Agency (ARPANSA), stated that scientific evidence indicated that it was *"highly unlikely"* that there was a link between the tumors and antennas.[iii]

A significant excess risk for adult brain tumours in electrical workers and those adults with occupational EMF exposure was reported by Kheifets *et al.*, 1995. (This is about the same size risk for lung cancer and second hand smoke (US DHHS, 2006).[iv] The three scientists involved in assessing the Californian Department of Health Services (DHS) EMF Program reviewed 29 epidemiological studies to come to the conclusion that they were *"inclined to believe that EMFs can cause some degree of increased risk of adult brain cancer"*.
(*Executive Summary of the California EMF Risk Evaluation For Policymakers And the Public*, The California Department of Health Services, June 2002).

Even though the result of our court case is quoted across the globe, it is public awareness that will change the way our systems operate. On being advised that the current guidelines do not address the cancer risk zealous residents in Wamberal, near Sydney bought attention to the often misunderstood guidelines in their fight against overhead powerlines. In July 2007 it was announced that Energy Australia is now under-grounding the new powerlines (which were originally to be overhead) in the high-density housing area. The community (www.wamberalactiongroup.com) is continuing to fight for some of the remainder of the powerlines to be under-grounded near a pre-school, primary school and high-school.

Lack of knowledge of the EMR/EMF issue often hampers the potential to prevent hundreds of thousands of people throughout the world from developing serious and fatal diseases. Too often the ELF EMF/RF EMF factor and the variables within it are never adequately addressed. Staff members often remain silent on suspected problems due to fear of losing employment and persecution. Legalities often prevent workplace situations from being adequately addressed. 'Whistleblowers' have a hard time under Australian laws.

Caution for Future Parents

Swedish male electrical switchyard workers when compared with non-exposed and socio-economic matched controls fathered more congenitally malformed children. After further testing on the switchyard workers, Dr Robert Becker commented: "The exposure to the electric-power frequency fields (50 Hz in Europe) produced abnormalities in chromosomes of the sperm of the switchyard workers, which resulted in birth defects in their children".[v]

(Refer to the work of Nordstrom and Nordensen *et al.* 1983, 1984, 1988). (Refer to Spitz *et al.* 1985 and Wilkins *et al.* 1988 for risk of brain tumour and nervous system cancers in children of male workers).

For maternal exposure: childhood leukaemia risk in the children of women who worked in industrial sewing machine factories. (Refer Van-Steensil Moll *et al.* 1985, Infante-Rivard 1995). As there is good evidence to suggest that much of childhood leukaemia involves a two-hit process, the first occurring *in utero* followed by a second in childhood, pregnant women must be cautious in their work situations and women's requests to transfer to duties away from areas with concentrated electrical equipment should be honored. (One of melatonin's many functions is the regulation of the sex hormones oestrogen and progesterone which are critical for full term pregnancies).

In the California Department of Health Services EMF Report the conclusions of the scientists were, in part, that all three were *"inclined to believe that EMFs can cause some degree of miscarriage"*. (*Executive Summary of the California EMF Risk Evaluation for Policymakers and the Public*, The California Department of Health Services, June 2002).

The California Public Utilities Commission who commissioned this report and paid over $7 million out of ratepayers funds has yet to review the findings in public forum.

ELF EMF and the variables within it, is still not regarded as the first and most important measurement to be taken in workplaces around the globe. Most of the public, and many employers, are unaware of this emerging health concern.

Additional Concerns

Workers are often concerned about masts and towers on their buildings so the focus is often on only testing for RF EMF measurements from the telecommunications antennas. Yet the equipment that runs these structures produces ELF EMF which is often significant and uncontrolled. These structures use electricity to generate the signal to transform the frequency.

Sub-stations on sites can deliver uncontrolled ELF EMF due to incorrect construction. ELF EMF from any source that is uncontrolled will find an outlet. Often significant, it can present in the wall next to an unfortunate individual or in a particular area in the workplace affecting even more unknowing victims. Transformers in buildings are often on the other side of a wall to employees or underneath them.

EMR measurements are often taken in workplaces when employees have already vacated the building (or at night) and the ELF EMF/RF EMF environment has changed. Of utmost importance is the need to investigate the ELF EMF/RF EMF factor in a real working environment. Limiting measurements to a single magnetic field reading does not account for all the variables. The electrical fields, presence of spikes, high frequency electrical transients, the position and continuing use of the elevators, the wiring in the building, and the location of sub-stations, transformers, switchgear and the equipment that generates the telecommunications equipment in relation to where individuals are located on a normal working day are only some of the factors that must be taken into account.

This information has the potential to: increase our knowledge in the interaction between humans and these fields; and impact on the lives of hundreds of thousands of women and men throughout the world in the quest to prevent cancer and cancer clusters. EMF has different effects in different combinations of exposure.

More comprehensive testing often results in sites being saved from demolition. 'Sick Building Syndrome' needs qualified EMR/EMF consultants to fully investigate the cause to put employees and employers at ease. Graham/Stetzer (GS) filters have been installed in schools with 'Sick Building Syndrome' and both staff and students reported improved health.

Milham and Morgan investigated a potential cancer cluster at La Quinta Middle School in La Quinta, California. They found:

"13 rooms in the school had very high levels of 'dirty

electricity' and the risk of cancer in these rooms was much higher than in electrically clean rooms. Teachers who never taught in these "dirty" rooms had a 1.8-fold risk of cancer while those who taught in these rooms had a 5.1-fold risk of cancer, and those who taught in these rooms and had been employed at this school for more than 10 years had a 7.1-fold risk of cancer".[vi]

(Refer Milham, S. and L. Morgan. 2007, *Teachers' Cancer Cluster at La Quinta Middle School.* http://www.buergerwelle.de/pdf/la_quinta_cancer_cluster.pdf).

Refer to Chapter Fourteen for how the use of filters in buildings, schools and homes is improving symptoms of many health disorders. Use of the Graham/Stetzer filters has reported reduced numbers of students needing inhalers for asthma and improved student behaviour associated with ADD/ADHD.

The occurrence of high magnetic fields is often brought to attention when newly installed office computers do not function properly due to electrical interference.

Machines and equipment can have high magnetic field emissions and some companies have taken serious steps to lessen the fields. Some workstations may emit high magnetic fields and manufacturers have adopted 2mG as the maximum emission value for ELF magnetic fields from computer monitors. Several multinational companies (including the World Bank) have specified magnetic fields of less than 2mG for their new building designs.

It is not only workplaces that can present with problems we must be mindful of our EMR/EMF environment in hospitals, schools, childcare centres and homes.

Most new housing estates have underground power, yet the feeder lines may be problematic. The feeder lines (which can yield high fields) to the underground power within an estate inspected were to run alongside children's bedrooms. The undergrounding of powerlines can significantly reduce magnetic fields, but not always. Underground powerlines must be configured correctly. Buried powerlines can generate lower magnetic fields than overhead powerlines because of their design, not because the earth eliminates the field. Two storey houses may have bedrooms parallel and very close to transformers on power poles outside their homes. Older houses may have higher fields as wiring codes have changed.

Electromagnetic fields can add to and strengthen each other, multiplying instead of dividing. It depends how the supply is configured. Faulty interior wiring, poor location of electrical system elements, unacceptable current flow on water and gas lines and electric heating coils in flooring can heighten EMF in the home and workplace. To lessen the effects of ELF EMF sub-stations need to be constructed properly and the presence of ground electrical return current on water piping addressed. Grounding errors and stray currents through water pipes can also interact with other fields. Electricity returns to earth via the easiest route – water pipes, the return wire, earth stake or an unfortunate person. Farmers have been dealing with stray current problems for decades. Ontario's Legislative Assembly has recently passed an Act to eliminate the problem of ground current in the state, striving to eliminate ground current problems in Ontario within ten years.

It is a matter of urgency that totally independent bodies with a clear charter be formed throughout the world so these cancer clusters be fully investigated. A totally independent body backed by strong advocacy, public awareness campaigns and a call for legislation changes would produce more effective results for potential victims of ELF EMF.

Electrohypersensitivity

Though there are still questions and more factors may be acknowledged in the interaction between electromagnetic energy and cellular biology in the future, electromagnetic sensitivity/electrohypersensitivity (EHS) is increasingly being acknowledged. EHS is recognised as a functional impairment in Sweden. The first WHO International Conference on EHS was in October 2004 in Prague.

At the Understanding Electrohypersensitivity Symposium in the Netherlands, December 2006, Michael Haas of the Institute of Building Biology in the Environment stated, "Electrosmog is an important reason for chronic tiredness, stress, aggression, depression, and other civilisation illnesses, even cancer. In the past 100 years the chance to get one of (these) illnesses increased from 1:1000 to 1:2!"[vii]

ELF EMF Interacting With Other Agents

In the early 1990s Liburdy and Harland reported that ELF EMF could interfere with the action of a hormone (melatonin) or drug (tamoxifen – *in vitro*). There is now also a growing body of literature showing that magnetic fields interact with known carcinogens or other toxic physical or chemical agents. Environmental agents which may not be genotoxic or carcinogenic by themselves, can contribute to cancer by increasing the genotoxic potential of other agents. "Very few environmental agents are known to promote carcinogens"[viii] yet "there is compelling evidence from laboratory studies that MFs enhance the effects of known carcinogens on cells".[ix] "The evidence supports the established mechanism by which magnetic fields can increase the lifetime of free radicals in the body and hence their ability to damage DNA".[x]

In their recent meta-analysis, Juutilainen *et al.* 2006 found the majority of studies reviewed were positive, suggesting that magnetic fields do interact with other chemical and physical exposures. The percentage of the 65 studies with positive effects was highest when the EMF exposure preceded the other exposure. The review collected 65 studies published between 1986 and 2002. (Refer Juutilainen *et al.* 2006 *Do extremely low frequency magnetic fields enhance the effects of environmental carcinogens? A meta-analysis of experimental studies* Int. J. Radiat. Biol., Vol. 82, No. 1, January 2006, pp. 1-12).

As the Juutilainen *et al.* 2006 study revealed that:

- the combined effects of toxic agents and ELF magnetic fields **together enhances damage** as compared to the toxic exposure alone, and

- the radical pair mechanism (oxidative damage due to free radicals) is cited as a good candidate to explain these results

reconsideration of exposure limits for ELF EMF is warranted based on this evidence.

(Refer to *Section 17 – Key Scientific Evidence and Public Health Policy Recommendations* – The BioInitiative Report).

i   Lamb 2002, p.3.
ii   Nader 2006
iii Nader 2006
iv Carpenter & Sage in Carpenter & Sage 2007, p.7
v   Becker 1990, p.211
vi Havas 2007, p.19
vii Haas in McLean 2007, p.8
viii Williams GM and Whysner J. in Morgan and Martin, p.19
ix Henshaw in R K Partnership Ltd 2007, p.58
x   Henshaw 2007, p.1-2

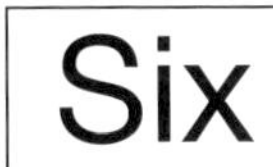

*I*t is now widely agreed that epidemiology consistently demonstrates an association between ELF magnetic fields and increased occurrence of childhood leukaemia. There are some particular papers which on their own could form the basis of a hypothesis that magnetic fields increase the risk of childhood leukaemia. Lupke *et al.* 2004 took human core blood and showed that magnetic fields release harmful reactive oxygen species (ROS). ROS includes free radicals and can damage DNA.

DNA damage due to free radicals is believed to be the initial oncostatic event in the majority of cancers (Cerutti *et al.* 1994). In addition to cancer, free radical damage in the central nervous system is a significant component of a variety of neurodegenerative diseases of the aged including Alzheimer's disease and Parkinson's disease.

Concern about this risk is mounting worldwide in regard to this emerging health issue. "For homes in the UK that have high background magnetic field levels, about one-third come from high-voltage overhead powerlines, one-third from faulty house wiring and equipment in the house and about one-third from electricity substations and mains voltage cables under the street".[i]

The SAGE Report

The UK SAGE (Stakeholder Advisory Group – formed in 2004 and funded equally by the Department of Health, the National Grid and CHILDREN with LEUKAEMIA) Interim Report in April 2007 identified the best-available option for obtaining significant exposure reduction is a restriction on new homes and schools close to existing lines, and on new lines close to existing homes and schools.

The SAGE Report also recommended:
- that electricity companies be encouraged to choose the optimal phasing (usually transposed phasing) for all new lines, and also

be encouraged to convert existing lines where possible and justifiable.

- guidance to electricians of recommended changes in wiring.
- information for householders on actions they can take to reduce fields from equipment in the home.
- more information be provided to members of the public about exposures and the actions they could take themselves to reduce exposures if they wished.

Where high magnetic fields as a result of house wiring are identified, the report recommends measures for remediation or removing exposure to such fields. Measures would include keeping beds, especially children's beds, away from meter cupboards, fuse boxes and transformers.

Considered a ground-breaking announcement, on July 18 2007 a report from a cross-party Inquiry of senior backbench MPs in the UK recommended that the Government ban new powerlines within 60 metres of existing homes and ban building new homes within 60 metres of existing powerlines. Over 220 MPs signed an Early Day Motion demanding that the Government supports CHILDREN WITH LEUKAEMIA's call for an immediate moratorium on new homes being built near power lines. Information packs to homeowners have also been called for on EMF measurements in the home.

The Inquiry has called for the introduction of precautionary measures following on from the Department of Health funded Draper Report. The Draper Report which was conducted by the Oxford Childhood Cancer Research Group in collaboration with National Grid and published in the *British Medical Journal* found that children living within 200m of high voltage power lines had a 70% higher risk of developing leukaemia than those living 600m or more away.

The Draper Report 2005 was the largest single study of childhood cancer and powerlines with roughly twice the number of children living close to powerlines than the next largest study (Feychting and Ahlbom 1993) as it examined 29,081 children with cancer – including 9700 with leukaemia – from the UK Cancer Registry. Children were aged 0-14 years and born in England and Wales, 1962-95. The authors concluded: "There is an association between childhood leukaemia and proximity of home address at birth to high voltage power lines, and the apparent risk extends to a greater distance than would have been expected from previous studies. About 4% of children in England and Wales live within 600 m of high voltage lines at birth… There is no accepted biological mechanism to explain the epidemiological results; indeed, the relation may be due to chance or confounding".

(Draper G, Vincent T, Kroll ME, Swanson J, 2005. *Childhood cancer in relation to distance from high voltage power lines in England and Wales: a case-control study.* BMJ; 330(7503):1290).

The Draper Report also found an increase of 23% in childhood leukaemia for those living between 200 and 600 metres from the powerlines. As magnetic fields are unlikely at this distance the theory of Professor Henshaw may indeed explain the mechanisation. Professor Denis Henshaw from Bristol University in the UK travels around the world lecturing on the phenomenon of corona ion emission from high voltage powerlines and how this "may explain an increased incidence of childhood leukaemia up to 600 metres from high voltage powerlines in England and Wales".

On commenting on the Draper Report Professor Henshaw states:

> "These latest findings not only strengthen further the evidence that children living in proximity to high voltage powerlines are at increased risk of childhood leukaemia, but in finding effects up to 600 metres away, they invoke electric field corona ion effects as a possible causal mechanism. The fact that this study has looked at the birth address is particularly important because the initial damage that may lead to leukaemia is thought to occur in-utero".[ii]

Professor Henshaw states corona ions are small electrically charged particles which when emitted from powerlines attach themselves to particles of air pollution. When such air pollution is inhaled it has a higher chance of being deposited in the lungs because of the increased electric charge carried by the corona ions. Once in the lungs such particles of air pollution can pass into the bloodstream reaching all body organs. As a result, there is greater uptake in the body of air pollution. Among other things, Professor Henshaw contends that this could lead to increased risk of lung cancer and leukaemia. A detailed description of his research and a more comprehensive summary of electromagnetic fields is available at: www.electric-fields.bris.ac.uk.

The Sage Report acknowledged the precautionary measures of Sweden and Denmark. It also acknowledged those of Italy, Switzerland, Israel, Netherlands and Slovenia (mostly applying to fields from power lines, almost applying to new lines or new homes near lines) and almost always applying to a specified list of locations such as homes, schools etc.

Lowenthal *et al.* (2007) reported that children raised for the first five years in home environments exposed to EMF within 300 meters of a high voltage power line have a five-fold (a 500 percent) increased risk of developing some kinds of cancers sometime in later life. For children from newborn to 15 years of age; it is a three-fold risk of developing cancer later in life. This study provides support for two important conclusions: **adult leukaemia is also associated with EMF exposure, and exposure during childhood increases risk of adult disease**. (*Summary for the Public* – The BioInitiative Report)

The Royal Commission on Environmental Pollution in July 2007 issued a short list of topics it is considering for its next study. The electromagnetic environment is currently on the list for submission. The Royal Commission on Environmental Pollution is an independent body, appointed by the Queen and funded by the government, which publishes in-depth reports on what it identifies as the crucial environmental issues facing the UK and the world with the full reports presented to Parliament.

A June 2007 report by the World Health Organisation (WHO) concluded that "provided that the health, social and economic benefits of electric power are not compromised, implementing very low-cost precautionary procedures to reduce exposure (to ELF EMF) is reasonable and warranted". (World Health Organisation (WHO) Environmental Health Criteria Monograph on Extremely Low Frequency Fields No. 238). This is seen as a very important step for enabling sensible legislation to be put in place.

Changing the Standards

As in the case with ELF EMF, existing standards for radiation frequency (RF EMF) and microwave (MW) radiation in most countries are still only designed to protect the public from just one aspect of effects, the 'gross' effects – the rise in body temperature – which is only seen with very high radiation intensities.

Compliance with the present standards does not mean protection from cancer or other disease risks. Like ELF EMF, there is no legislation in place to protect the public in regard to RF EMF in most countries. "The scientific studies on which our standards are set were observations made in the 1970s of behavioural change in primates exposed to heat-emitting devices".[iii]

EMR across the non-ionising spectrum includes the fields from electricity (ELF EMF) and the fields from communications equipment (RF EMF/MW). Because microwaves (MW) are also used for communications RF and microwave emissions MW overlap considerably. (Refer to Appendix A and Appendix B).

ELF EMF and RF EMF often have overlapping exposures that occur in daily life. Both ELF EMF and RF EMF exposures have been shown to cause similar effects, for example, cause cells to generate stress proteins, a universal sign of distress in plant, animal and human cells.

Authorities around the world still keep in place guidelines based on the premise that these fields have to be very intense to produce visible effects such as electric shock and burns. The recognised biophysical mechanisms being that external ELF magnetic fields induce electric fields and currents in the body which, at very high field strengths, cause nerve and muscle stimulation and changes in nerve cell excitability in the central nervous system.

The premise that humans can detect these invisible fields is forcing long-standing beliefs in regard to ELF EMF to be discarded. Arguments that ELF EMF cannot affect biological systems do not represent the current spectrum of scientific opinion. As far back as 1992 Morgan and Nair stated: "Leading researchers in bioelectromagnetics agree that ELF EMF have cellular, immune, and neuroendocrine effects despite relatively low energies".[iv]

The current guidelines for Australia are:
- 1000mG for the general public (24 hour); and
- 5000mG for occupational exposure (8 hour).

This has been a voluntary exposure standard with no enforcement or verification program by either State or Federal governments.

Professor Andrew Wood is the chairman of the ARPANSA Working Group who is currently developing the new ELF standard for Australia expected to be completed late 2008.

The latest progress report on the new ELF standard is:

- 3000mG for the general public; and
- 15000mG for occupational exposure.

Effects occur at non-thermal (or low-intensity) exposure levels thousands of times below the levels that federal authorities/agencies deem to be safe for the public.

Those who are setting the exposure standards are protecting us against what damage heating causes. This is important. The problem is that other evidence – that shows lower intensity fields are important if they contain information content that disturbs how cells normally function – has not been addressed as yet. It appears it is the information conveyed by electromagnetic radiation at intensities that do not cause heating that can also cause biological changes of not yet fully explored consequences.

ELF EMF may be eventually "elevated in the hierarchy" of IARC categories from a 'possible' carcinogen (Category 2B) to a 'probable' carcinogen (Category 2A) because of the mounting scientific evidence.

The view expressed by Professor Philip Jennings in his submission to the Australian Inquiry into Electromagnetic Radiation (2001) should be the underlying premise when attending to public health policies in regard to EMR/EMF:

> Our society's experience with ionising radiation should persuade us to take great care … The original standard set for ionising radiation protection … has proven to be quite inappropriate and as further research has been performed and evaluated **the public limit has been reduced by nearly a factor of a thousand**. This could also happen with EMR. We are still in the infancy of EMR research and we should learn from the mistakes we made with ionising radiation and introduce a principle of prudent avoidance or ALARA.[v]

The recently released *scientific review* The BioInitiative Report is now challenging the EMF power structure to set much stricter standards for powerlines – **1000 times less than the standards abided by most countries**. RF EMF is also addressed calling for much stricter standards for mobile phones and cordless phones.

Highly-respected and award-winning Associate Professor Olle Johansson MD Department of Neuroscience of the Karolinska Institute, Stockholm, Sweden has observed that: "cellular damage in people with EHS closely resembles radiation damage found in people exposed to UV-light or ionizing radiation".[vi]

Olle Johansson in *Section 8 – Evidence for Effects on the Immune System* – of The BioInitiative Report comments that today no-one would consider having a radioactive wrist watch with glowing digits (as you could in the 1950s), having your children's shoes fitted in a strong X-ray machine (as you could in the 1940s), keeping radium in open trays on your desk (as scientists could in the 1930s), or x-raying each other at your garden party (as physicians did in the 1920s). Safety measures are now in place when performing and receiving x-rays. The cardinal principles of radiation protection that are currently enforced for ionising radiation are: time, distance and shielding. It would be sensible to also apply this to ELF EMF.

Radiation was the first known proven cause of cancer. It was many years before Western scientists acknowledged radiation sickness and radiation related cancers from the ionising radiation of the atomic bombs on Hiroshima and Nagasaki. A plausible mechanism was required and it took many years of research to identify the mechanism through which the radioactive material released ionising radiation that produced free radicals, which in turn caused single and double strand breakage of DNA and cancer.

As far back as 1966 biological health effects were reported in Soviet sub-station workers. Epidemiology compares large groups that have been exposed to an agent with other groups that have not been exposed, e.g., smokers versus non-smokers. Everyone is exposed to ELF EMF and this enables the problem to be masked: risk may be under-estimated as it is hard to gather a truly unexposed comparison group.

Controversial associations between toxic agents and their affect on disease, for example, x-rays, chronic use of tobacco and asbestos are never welcomed. Sir Richard Doll was, at first, heavily criticised for his contention on the link between cigarette smoke and lung cancer. It has taken over 40 years of research and advocacy for the dangers of tobacco smoking to be acknowledged by governments and another decade for measures and legislation to be instigated to protect the public. More recently, the dangers associated with asbestos are being addressed and safety measures are being implemented to protect the workers handling asbestos.

Dr Cherry maintained that the progressive elevation of household electromagnetic fields has contributed to a significant amount of the increase in leukaemia, breast cancer, brain tumour and other cancers in the adult population over the period from about 1920 onwards. He showed that occupational studies also provide strong and consistent evidence that EMR/EMF occupational exposure is causally related to increases in leukaemia, breast cancer and brain tumours.

The use of electricity is central to our way of living: not all the population engages in the smoking of tobacco or have been exposed to the hazards associated with asbestos. To correct the problems of the current electrical systems and wiring already in place can, in some, but certainly not all cases, be an expensive process. Acknowledging the ill-effects from an agent that we all pay for, that is able to compromise the immune system and therefore set the body up for serious and fatal disease might open the floodgates and cost billions in lawsuits. Some medical legal experts have seen this possibility and suggest the scale of the litigation would dwarf the asbestos experience.

No matter what side of the argument one's opinion sits on in regard to the ELF EMF issue, surely we must do all we can as a civilisation to protect the physical and mental health of the people within it. Never before has science met such a challenge that questions effects at core bodily processes. A toxic agent which totally governs our way of living that has the potential to change our fundamental bodily processes at a core level with such severe consequences can have great resistance in addressing its consequences.

Something that even whispers at this conclusion should be enough to encourage those who are entrusted to protect us to act in our best interests to ensure the health of people and the prosperity of more generations to come.

The effect of an environmental pollutant whether it has been DDT, lead, tobacco smoking or asbestos, is often observed long before the mechanism of action is understood. These toxic agents had their experts who stated that the results were inconclusive or contradictory or unproven until the mechanism of action was identified.

Even though we are now surrounded by an unprecedented level of artificial electromagnetic energy – electromagnetic fields and electromagnetic radiation – that has no precedent in the history of civilisation there has been extensive and rigorous testing in regard to ELF EMF that still continues to this day.

Although it is not necessary to identify a biological mechanism for classifying a causal effect (Hill 1965) further research is being conducted to clarify what exact processes are involved. What remains to be known in terms of mechanisms is unlikely to significantly change what is already known. Plausible biological mechanisms are already identified that can reasonably account for most biological effects. It is not necessary for public policy makers to wait until all the scientific facts are in, enough is known – and has been for many years – to justify minimising exposures. Although a lot is known about cancer the mechanism of cancer in general is still not known.

As far back as the 1990s, it was acknowledged that the research is as conclusive as the data relating to cigarette smoking and cancer. Dr Thomas C Erren MPH, Institute and Policlinic for Occupational and Social Medicine, University of Cologne, Germany stated in 1997:

> "There are more epidemiologic studies that link cancer to ELF EMF than to environmental tobacco smoke (ETS)".[vii]

i   Powerwatch 2007, p.1
ii   Henshaw 2005, p.1
iii The Parliament of the Commonwealth of Australia 2001, p.xxi
iv   Erren in Stevens, Wilson, Anderson, 1977, p.704
v   The Parliament of the Commonwealth of Australia 2001, p.32
vi   Johansson in McLean 2007, p.9
vii Erren in Stevens, Wilson, Anderson, 1977, p.729

The formation of the International Commission for Electromagnetic Safety (ICEMS) in Italy in 2003 is seeking to implement measures to protect the public.

Promoting independent research in bioelectromagnetics, the International Commission on Electromagnetic Safety is a not-for-profit group of world-leading concerned scientists striving for the implementation of worldwide legislation in regard to EMR: ELF EMF and RF EMF (0-300 GHz).

Previously supporting public opposition to two high power transmission lines running through the village of Contrada San Vitale, that led to their removal, Dr Sandro D'Allessandro, Mayor of Benevento, sponsored the ICEMS EMF workshop in Benevento, Italy in February 2006. This workshop, dedicated to the late Australian born Dr Ross Adey, invited participants from twelve countries: Brazil, Canada, China, Israel, Italy, Poland, Russia, Sweden, Taiwan, Turkey, United Kingdom and the United States of America.

In September 2006 after several months of debate, thirty-one world-respected scientists signed the Benevento Resolution to advise the public and the scientific community of their strong belief that there are adverse health effects affirming the Catania Resolution adopted in 2002.

Particular points of interest from the Benevento Resolution in regard to ELF EMF and RF EMF are:

The Benevento Resolution scientists resolved that "epidemiological and laboratory studies that show increased risks for cancers and other diseases from occupational exposures to EMF cannot be ignored, and independent, transparent examination of the evidence is needed". [i]

Point 3: "there is evidence that present sources of funding bias the analysis and interpretation of research findings towards rejection of evidence of possible public health risks". [ii]

Point 4: "arguments that weak (low intensity) EMF cannot affect biological systems do not represent the current spectrum of scientific opinion". [iii] Weak (low intensity) refers to extremely low frequency (ELF) EMF.

Point 5: "Based on our review of the science, biological effects can occur from exposures to both extremely low frequency fields (ELF EMF) and radiation frequency fields (RF EMF). Epidemiological and *in vivo*, as well as *in vitro*, experimental evidence demonstrates that exposure to some ELF EMF can increase cancer risk in children and induce other health problems in both children and adults…". [iv]

Point 5: "…Further, there is accumulating epidemiological evidence indicating an increased brain tumor risk from long term use of mobile phone phones, the first RF EMF that has started to be comprehensively studied". [v]

Point 5: "Epidemiological and laboratory studies that show increased risk for cancers and other diseases from occupational exposures to EMF cannot be ignored". [vi]

Point 6.1: "Promote alternatives to wireless communication systems". [vii]

Point 6.1: "Design cellular phones that meet safer performance specifications, including radiating away from the head". [viii]

Point 6.1: "… place power lines underground in the vicinity of populated areas, only siting them in residential neighborhoods as a last resort". [ix]

Point 6.2: "Inform the population of the potential risks of cell phone and cordless phone use. Advise consumers to limit wireless calls and use a land line for long conversations". [x]

Point 6.3: "Limit cell phone and cordless phone use by young children and teenagers to the lowest possible level and urgently ban telecom companies from marketing to them". [xi]

Point 6.5: "Protect workers from EMF generating equipment, through access restrictions and EMF shielding of both individuals and physical structures". [xii]

Point 6.6: "Plan communications antenna and tower locations to minimize human exposure…".[xiii]

Point 6.7: "Designate wireless-free zones …".[xiv]

i   2006 Benevento Resolution, www.icems.eu
ii   2006 Benevento Resolution, www.icems.eu
iii   2006 Benevento Resolution, www.icems.eu
iv   2006 Benevento Resolution, www.icems.eu
v   2006 Benevento Resolution, www.icems.eu
vi   2006 Benevento Resolution, www.icems.eu
vii   2006 Benevento Resolution, www.icems.eu
viii   2006 Benevento Resolution, www.icems.eu
ix   2006 Benevento Resolution, www.icems.eu
x   2006 Benevento Resolution, www.icems.eu
xi   2006 Benevento Resolution, www.icems.eu
xii   2006 Benevento Resolution, www.icems.eu
xiii   2006 Benevento Resolution, www.icems.eu
xiv   2006 Benevento Resolution, www.icems.eu

The BENEVENTO RESOLUTION is as follows:

The International Commission for Electromagnetic Safety (ICEMS) held an international conference entitled *"The Precautionary EMF Approach: Rationale, Legislation and Implementation"*, hosted by the City of Benevento, Italy, on February 22, 23 & 24, 2006. The meeting was dedicated to W. Ross Adey, M.D. (1922-2004). The scientists at the conference endorsed and extended the 2002 Catania Resolution and resolved that:

1. More evidence has accumulated suggesting that there are adverse health effects from occupational and public exposures to electric, magnetic and electromagnetic fields, or EMF[i] at current exposure levels. What is needed, but not yet realized, is a comprehensive, independent and transparent examination of the evidence pointing to this emerging, potential public health issue.

2. Resources for such an assessment are grossly inadequate despite the explosive growth of technologies for wireless communications as well as the huge ongoing investment in power transmission.

3. There is evidence that present sources of funding bias the analysis and interpretation of research findings towards rejection of evidence of possible public health risks.

4. Arguments that weak (low intensity) EMF cannot affect biological systems do not represent the current spectrum of scientific opinion.

5. Based on our review of the science, biological effects can occur from exposures to both extremely low frequency fields (ELF EMF) and radiation frequency fields (RF EMF). Epidemiological and in vivo as well as in vitro experimental evidence demonstrates that exposure to some ELF EMF can increase cancer risk in children and induce other health problems in both children and adults. Further, there is accumulating epidemiological evidence indicating an increased brain tumor risk from long term use of mobile phones, the first RF EMF that has started to be comprehensively studied. Epidemiological and laboratory studies that show increased risks for cancers and other diseases from occupational exposures to EMF cannot be ignored. Laboratory studies on cancers and other diseases have reported that hypersensitivity to EMF may be due in part to a genetic predisposition.

6. We encourage governments to adopt a framework of guidelines for public and occupational EMF exposure that reflect the Precautionary Principle[ii] – as some nations have already done. Precautionary strategies should be based on design and performance standards and may not necessarily define numerical thresholds because such thresholds may erroneously be interpreted as levels below which no adverse effect can occur. These strategies should include:

- 6.1 Promote alternatives to wireless communication systems, e.g., use of fiber optics and coaxial cables; design cellular phones that meet safer performance specifications, including radiating away from the head; preserve existing land line phone networks; place power lines underground in the vicinity of populated areas, only siting them in residential neighborhoods as a last resort;

- 6.2 Inform the population of the potential risks of cell phone and cordless phone use. Advise consumers to limit wireless calls and use a land line for long conversations.

- 6.3 Limit cell phone and cordless phone use by young children and teenagers to the lowest possible level and urgently ban telecom companies from marketing to them.

- 6.4 Require manufacturers to supply hands-free kits (via speaker phones or ear phones), with each cell phone and cordless phone.

- 6.5 Protect workers from EMF generating equipment, through access restrictions and EMF shielding of both individuals and physical structures.

- 6.6 Plan communications antenna and tower locations to minimize human exposure. Register mobile phone base stations with local planning agencies and use computer mapping technology to inform the public on possible exposures. Proposals for city-wide wireless access systems (e.g. Wi-Fi, WIMAX, broadband over cable or power-line or equivalent technologies) should require public review of potential EMF exposure and, if installed, municipalities should ensure this information is available to all and updated on a timely basis.

- 6.7 Designate wireless-free zones in cities, in public buildings (schools, hospitals, residential areas) and, on public transit, to permit access by persons who are hypersensitive to EMF.

7. ICEMS[iii] is willing to assist authorities in the development of an EMF research agenda. ICEMS encourages the development of clinical and epidemiological protocols for investigations of geographical clusters of persons with reported allergic reactions and other diseases or sensitivities to EMF, and document the effectiveness of preventive interventions. ICEMS encourages scientific collaboration and reviews of research findings.

---

i   EMF, in this resolution, refers to zero to 300 GHz.

ii   The Precautionary Principle states when there are indications of possible adverse effects, though they remain uncertain, the risks from doing nothing may be far greater than the risks of taking action to control these exposures. The Precautionary Principle shifts the burden of proof from those suspecting a risk to those who discount it.

iii International Commission for Electromagnetic Safety

$\mathscr{T}$he BioInitiative Report was released on August 31, 2007. This ***scientific review*** of more than 2000 studies produced by an international working group of world-leading and widely respected scientists, researchers and public health policy professionals concludes that there are many biological effects at levels that are well below current limits and that the existing safety limits are inadequate to protect public health.

The BioInitiative Report states "it appears it is the **INFORMATION** conveyed by electromagnetic radiation (rather than heat) that causes biological changes – some of these biological changes may lead to loss of wellbeing, disease and even death".[i] (*Summary for the Public*).

The BioInitiative Report clearly states: "**the scientific evidence is sufficient to warrant regulatory action for ELF; and it is substantial enough to warrant preventative actions for RF**".[ii]

Conclusions in *Summary for the Public* of The BioInitiative Report include:

ELF EMF

- there is little doubt that exposure to ELF causes childhood leukaemia.

- there is some evidence that other childhood cancers may be related to ELF exposure but not enough studies have been done.

- children who have leukaemia and are in recovery have poorer survival rates if their ELF exposure at home (or where they are recovering) is between 1mG and 2mG in one study; over 3mG in another study.

- studies of human breast cancer cells and some animal studies show that ELF is likely to be a risk factor for breast cancer. There is supporting evidence for a link between breast cancer and exposure to ELF that comes from cell and animal studies, as well as studies of human breast cancers.

- alzheimer's disease is a disease of the nervous system. There is strong evidence that long-term exposure to ELF is a risk factor for Alzheimer's disease.

- oxidative stress through the action of free radical damage to DNA is a plausible biological mechanism for cancer and diseases that involve damage from ELF to the central nervous system.

RF EMF

- there is little doubt that electromagnetic fields emitted by cell phones and cordless phones use affect electrical activity in the brain.

- people who have used a cell phone for ten years or more have higher rates of malignant brain tumor and acoustic neuromas. It is worse if the cell phone has been used primarily on one side of the head.

- people who have used a cordless phone for ten years or more have higher rates of malignant brain tumor and acoustic neuromas. It is worse if the cordless phone has been used primarily on one side of the head.

ELF EMF and RF EMF

- both ELF and RF exposure can be considered genotoxic (will damage DNA) under certain conditions of exposure including exposure levels that are lower than existing safety limits.

- very low level ELF and RF exposures can cause cells to produce stress proteins, meaning that the cell recognizes ELF and RF exposures as harmful.

- there is substantial evidence that ELF and RF can cause inflammatory reactions, allergy reactions and change normal immune function at levels allowed by current public safety standards.

- medical conditions are successfully treated using EMFs at levels below current public safety standards, proving another way that the body recognises and corresponds to low-intensity EMF signals. Otherwise, these medical treatments could not work. The FDA has approved EMFs as medical treatment devices so is clearly aware of this paradox.

The BioInitiative Report recommends that new ELF limits are warranted based on a public health analysis of the overall existing scientific evidence.

Also included in The BioInitiative working group's report are recommendations:

- that it is no longer acceptable to build new power lines and electrical facilities that place people in ELF environments that have been determined to be risky – these levels are in the 2 to 4mG range.

- while new ELF limits are being developed and implemented, a reasonable approach would be a **1mG** planning limit for habitable space adjacent to all new or upgraded power lines and a **2mG** limit for all other new construction.

- the occupation of seamstress deserves attention in future studies as seamstresses are in fact one of the most highly MF exposed occupations with exposure levels generally above 10mG (1.0μT) over a significant proportion of the workday. They also have been consistently found to be at higher risk of Alzheimer's disease and (female) breast cancer.

This next recommendation is based on the assumption that "a higher burden of protection is required for children who cannot protect themselves, and who are at risk for childhood leukemia at rates that are traditionally high enough to trigger regulatory action":[iii]

- a 1mG limit be established for existing habitable space for children and/or women who are pregnant (because of the possible link between childhood leukemia and *in utero* exposure to ELF).

Section 11 Evidence for Childhood Cancers (Leukemia) states: "the balance of evidence suggests that childhood leukemia is associated with exposure to power frequency EMFs either during early life or pregnancy".[iv] Professor Kundi further states: "Up to 80% of childhood leukemia may be caused by exposure to power frequency EMF".[v]

The BioInitiative Report brings attention to the fact that "traditional public health and epidemiological determinations do not require a proven mechanism before inferring a causal link between EMFs exposure and disease".[vi] "Plausible biological mechanisms are already identified that can reasonably account for most biological effects reported for exposure to RF and ELF at low-intensity levels ...".[vii]

The European Environmental Agency endorses The BioInitiative Report.

The Breast Cancer Fund – USA – supports The BioInitiative Report statement that the scientific evidence is sufficient to warrant regulatory action for ELF EMF and is substantial enough to warrant preventive actions for RF EMF. The Breast Cancer Fund – USA – also states that based on the scientific evidence set forth in The BioInitiative Report and a growing body of additional research, exposure limits for electromagnetic radiation should be set at the federal level.

For a more in-depth condensed summary of the EMR/EMF issue, its history, studies and areas recommended for future study refer to The BioInitiative Report: *A Rationale for a Biologically-based Public Exposure Standard for Electromagnetic Fields (ELF and RF)* at www.bioinitiative.org.

i   Sage in Carpenter and Sage (eds) 2007, p.6
ii   Sage in Carpenter and Sage (eds) 2007, p.21
iii Sage in Carpenter and Sage (eds) 2007, p.22
iv   Kundi in Carpenter and Sage (eds) 2007, p.14
v   Kundi in Carpenter and Sage (eds) 2007, p.14
vi   Sage in Carpenter and Sage (eds) 2007, p.19
vii Sage in Carpenter and Sage (eds) 2007 p.19

Nine

$\mathscr{I}$n December 2006 the majority of staff left the ABC TV studios in Toowong, Brisbane, Australia after a cancer cluster had been determined. Since 1994, seventeen staff working at this workplace have been diagnosed with breast cancer. In the *Breast Cancer at the ABC Toowong Queensland: Third Progress Report –* Independent Review and Scientific Investigation Panel dated 21 December 2006, after discounting all other factors (including genetics, lifestyle, and toxic agents) the workplace was acknowledged as the problem. The many experts engaged could not find the problem. No agent could be found to be responsible for the breast cancer cluster.

Dr Geza Benke, in the ABC report states: "…Ionising radiation is the only known environmental exposure that is known with certainty to increase breast cancer risk".[i] Point 3 a. of the ABC report stated above states that there is no documented history of the use of ionising radiation on the site.

The EMC Technologies report B050401 of 2 May 2005, Point 4.3 states: a specific request had been made by staff to measure the fields next to a cable tray running in a wall near Jo-Anne Youngleson's desk in the newsroom general area. RF field levels were taken as the EMC Technologies Report focused on radio frequency – RF.

Being a wiring cable tray, the wiring current flow would have emitted ELF EMF.

Many months later, Dr Geza Benke finally recommended ELF EMF measurements. Dr Benke in Point 3.c page 12 of the *Breast Cancer at the ABC Toowong Queensland:Third Progress Report* states:

> "ELF exposure has not been measured in the TV building. Given the high concentration of communications equipment in many of the workstations in this building, exposure is expected to be higher than in a normal office environment. The power requirements of the ABC Toowong site are clearly

high, given that it has its own sub-station. Thus the power intensive sources and high power frequency currents required for high ELF exposures are present on the site."[ii]

EMC Technologies had previously conducted all other testing of fields (RF EMF) at this site. The Australian Government's ARPANSA, measured the ELF EMF on December 18 2006.

After conducting measurements, Mr Ken Karipidis from ARPANSA in completing his assessment states: "In general these measurements indicate that the levels are lower than what is usually encountered in a normal office environment".[iii] Mr Karipidis from ARPANSA reported in the Third Progress Report Page 13, that the measurements were 'averaged': "The average magnetic field was about 1mG".[iv]

'Averages' can dilute high measurements in that if one area in the room measured 0mG and another area measured 26mG 'averaging' dilutes the fields where the problem presented.

The ABC TV station where the breast cancer cluster occurred produced a two-part story on the program *Australian Story*, which aired in Australia – *Part One* on Monday 12 March 2006 and *Part Two* on Monday 19 March 2006. In *Part Two*, Professor Armstrong acknowledged: "There's evidence to suggest in some populations with high shift work that the risk of breast cancer can be up to about two times higher than what it is in the general population. It's certainly nothing like the sixfold increase in risk that we observed on the ABC site".[v] Professor Armstrong stated: "We felt that extremely low frequency electromagnetic energy was a possible issue". [vi] This means ELF EMF.

The ARPANSA ELF Report indicates that three ABC volunteers wore data loggers for four hours to determine the practicality of using the EMDEX 11 instruments for this purpose. The ARPANSA ELF Report February 2007 states on page 2, point 2, that **"it is unknown how representative their work patterns (volunteers) were of the women suffering health effects"**. The ARPANSA survey consisted of a two hour walk taking spot measurements around the studios. There is no mention of the measurements of the ELF EMF next to a cable tray running in a wall near Jo-Anne Youngleson's desk in the newsroom area being specifically addressed in the ARPANSA February 2007 report. Media reports often referred to 'that particular desk" that concerned staff.

Mr John Lincoln, the community representative on a working group for the ELF EMF standard run by ARPANSA appeared on *Part Two* of the *Australian Story* program. On commenting on the fact that ARPANSA only did spot measurements at the ABC, he made the following statement:

> "From what I've seen of the ABC testing, I'm not that happy with it because spot testing is not good enough. A minimum of 48 hours is needed for a thorough test and in some cases I would leave a data longer for four or five days. From the results that Dr Armstrong has been given I think I would arrive at the same conclusions he has had. My question is, are they comprehensive enough? Do they really cover the situation?"[vii]

A more recent Japanese study found high magnetic fields in a bedroom – exposed to 4mG or more – could increase the risk of childhood leukaemia by up to nearly five times. Week long measurements as well as spot measurements were taken. The measurements were also taken close to time of diagnosis. (Kabuto *et al.*2005).

We will never know what specific ELF EMF the breast cancer victims were exposed to. The impact of the loss of more detailed ELF EMF information in regard to this breast cancer cluster is enormous.

Interviewed on the Australia programme '*Nine with David and Kim*' on August 7, 2007 and questioned on this breast cancer cluster and the frustration of some of the women who felt the proper investigations were not carried out before all the equipment was taken out Professor Armstrong stated: "It is very important to do the investigations properly and indeed we did have a problem with the ABC with the fairly quick decision to remove people from the site, it did mean that some of the measurements we wanted to do were not complete and I do understand how the women feel in that respect, they don't feel that it's been done satisfactorily…".

Inadequate ELF EMF testing often prevents the association between breast cancer in women and ELF EMF being officially acknowledged as stronger. The three scientists involved in the Californian Department of Health Services (DHS) EMF Program reported: "*to one degree or another they are inclined to believe that EMFs do not cause an increased risk of breast cancer*".

(*Executive Summary of the California EMF Risk Evaluation For Policymakers And the Public*, The California Department of Health Services, June 2002).

More detailed ELF EMF information from this particular breast cancer cluster may have revealed why there have been inconsistencies in the breast cancer studies.

There is evidence of spikes in the ARPANSA graph. Further testing for 'dirty electricity'/'dirty power' – a newer metric exposure – may have also revealed that 'dirty electricity' – high frequency transients – also played a part in creating this breast cancer cluster. 'Dirty electricity' generated by electrical equipment in the building is distributed throughout the building on the electrical wiring travelling along the electrical distribution system in and between buildings and through the ground. Humans and conducting objects in contact with the ground become part of the circuit.

As far back as 1997 it was observed that: "The results of the Probe Experiment are consistent with other indications suggesting that transients produced by rapid electric and/or magnetic field onset/offset might be a critical feature producing melatonin suppression".[viii] Henshaw & Reiter (2005) found that effects on melatonin disruption were more pronounced when switching or transients of magnetic fields were present which concurred with other findings.

i   Benke in Armstrong 2006, p.12
ii   Armstrong 2006, p.12
iii   Armstrong 2006, p.13
iv   Armstrong 2006, p.13
v   abc.net.au/austory/content/2007/s1876734.htm 2007, p.6
vi   abc.net.au/austory/content/2007/s1876734.htm 2007, p.6
vii   abc.net.au/austory/content/2007/s1876734.htm 2007, p.6
viii   Rogers, Reiter, Orr in Stevens, Wilson, Anderson, ed, 1997, p.463

Ten

$\mathscr{B}$reast cancer is the number one cancer in women throughout the world. The role of man-made toxic agents must be vigorously researched as only "approximately 5 to 7 percent of all breast cancer is attributable to inherited mutations in two different genes: BRCA1 and BRCA2".[i]

Once again, as in their controversial study linking ELF EMF and childhood cancer in their study of 1979, the work of Dr Nancy Wertheimer and Ed Leeper is pivotal in the area of breast cancer.

Wertheimer and Leeper (1982) were the first to see a magnetic field-breast cancer connection in their 1982 study of residential magnetic field exposures of adults. Even though this paper was of overall cancer risk in adults and was not designed to look specifically at breast cancer they discovered a nearly threefold increase among women younger than 55 who lived near power lines, indicating that magnetic field exposure had accelerated development and growth of breast cancer.

(Refer Wertheimer N, Leeper E. *Adult cancer related to electrical wires near the home.* Int J Epidemiol 1982 11:345-355).

The first evidence of increased breast cancer risk in women in electrical occupations was reported by Loomis *et al.* 1994. This study which raised many questions used U.S. national death certificate information for women (which is not optimal) who had died of breast cancer from 1985-1989 and their occupational titles. The intriguing findings – women in traditional electrical occupations were found to have a nearly 40% higher mortality from breast cancer – were found to be broadly consistent with the hypothesis that exposure to ELF EMF causes breast cancer among women. Also, twice the expected number of breast cancer deaths was observed for female electrical workers aged 45 to 54 compared to women working at other jobs.

(Refer Loomis DP, Savitz DA, Ananth CV. *Breast cancer mortality among female electrical workers in the United States.* Journal of National Cancer Inst 1994; 86:921–925).

Further research has reported that exposure to extremely low frequency electromagnetic fields (ELF EMF) may indeed play a crucial role in the breast cancer risk equation.

In 1997 the findings of thirty-eight scientists were published in *The Melatonin Hypothesis: Breast Cancer and the Use of Electric Power*. The 'Melatonin Hypothesis' proposed: "exposure to 'light at night' and/or EMF may disrupt the function of the pineal gland and its primary hormone melatonin and that this disruption lowers melatonin production, a consequence that may lead to an increase in the long-term risk of breast cancer".[ii]

A protective association between melatonin and breast cancer development is now supported. Higher levels of melatonin are associated with a lower risk of breast cancer. In fact, it is the area of breast cancer where the cancer-suppressing effects of melatonin are most supportive.

As melatonin is a known cancer-suppressing agent any factor that depresses its production, secretion or actions may contribute to an increased cancer risk. In regard to ELF EMF magnetic fields have been shown to suppress the function of the pineal gland and decrease the production and release of melatonin by the pineal gland. A reduction in the pineal gland's production of melatonin would increase susceptibility to sex hormone-related cancers. Breast cancer is a hormone-related cancer: high levels of sex-hormones can raise the risk of breast cancer.

"Lack of melatonin can reasonably be anticipated to be a human carcinogen"[iii] as stated by C.J. Portier of the National Institute of Environmental Health Sciences (NIEHS/NIH) – an Institute within the National Toxicology Program.

Further ELF EMF laboratory research has also shown:
- ELF EMF of **12mG can block the ability of melatonin** to inhibit human breast cancer cells.
- ELF EMF of **12mG can block the ability of tamoxifen** to control the growth of human breast cancer cells.

As fields of 12mG can be encountered in workplaces and also in situations where older/incorrect wiring presents these effects have **enormous implications**.

Oestrogen dominance is indicated in playing a role in breast cancer with melatonin playing a vital role in breast cancer protection. As two thirds of all breast cancer are oestrogen-dependant (growth is promoted by oestrogen) lessening exposure to high fields of ELF EMF appears critical for oestrogen-dependent breast cancer. More funding in this area also has the potential to lead to successful noninvasive treatments for breast cancer.

For a concise summary of the controversial findings, the studies and the acknowledgement and calibre of the scientists involved in this area and the '12mG effect', refer to www.microwavenews.com article *When Enough is Never Enough: A Reproducible Effect at 2mG-12mG*" by Louis Slesin PhD.

Louis Slesin comments in this article that the important papers by Robert Liburdy, Carl Blackman and Masimo Ishido documenting the 12mG effect on melatonin and tamoxifen were not included in the recent World Health Organization's EMF Project – a 365-page document with over 1000 references.

Dr Cherry

Canada has one of the highest rates of breast cancer in the world. As far back as July 1999, Dr Cherry presented a paper *Electromagnetic Radiation and Breast Cancer* at the World Breast Cancer Conference in Ottawa, Canada.

Dr Cherry stated studies have shown significant increases in male and female breast cancer from exposure to EMR from ELF EMF to RF EMF, as with leukaemia and brain tumour.

Dr Cherry maintained:

- "breast tissue is very sensitive to free radical damage and hence to melatonin reduction."[vi]
- "there is a tendency for higher rates in pre-menopausal women and those with estrogen-receptor positive breast cancer (ER+), and for black women".[v]
- EMR is especially active in initiating and/or accelerating oestrogen-receptor positive (rich in oestrogen receptors) breast cancer.
- women under 50 years of age have more EMR induced breast cancer than other women in the same age range.

"Breast cancer is the leading cause of death in women between 40 and 50 years of age".[vi]

Breast Cancer in Men

The link between ELF EMF and breast cancer became more prominent due to the unusual occurrence of breast cancer in males, a disease normally so rare, that only about one case is diagnosed in every one hundred thousand men each year.

Most of the studies involving measurements of occupational magnetic fields had been limited to men. "…**An association between ELF EMF and breast cancer is supported in men**".[vii]

Female breast cancer has multiple risk factors which presents difficulties in strengthening the ELF EMF breast cancer association. The more risk factors the easier it can be to discount the exact cause. Additional factors such as reproductive risk factors (for example, age at menarche, number of births, and age at menopause) are not relevant to men.

A cluster of male breast cancer in one area would suggest a single dominant risk factor in those cases. An occupational study was conducted by Milham (2004), who investigated a cluster of male breast cancer in a small group of men who worked in a basement office in a multi-storey office building. Their office was adjacent to an electrical switchgear room that generated high magnetic fields in their workspace (50+mG). This risk of male breast cancer in this group was increased about 100-fold.[viii]

Further research – An ELF EMF prostate cancer link is also proposed as like breast cancer, prostate cancer is also a hormone-dependent cancer. Most prostate cancers are testosterone-dependent.

The BioInitiative Report

The BioInitiative Report of August 31 2007 contributed to by an international working group of world-leading and widely respected scientists, researchers and public health policy professionals states:

> **"there is sufficient evidence from in vitro and animal studies, from human biomarker studies, from occupational and light-at-night studies, and a single longitudinal study with appropriate collection of urine**

samples to conclude that high MF exposure may be a risk factor for breast cancer".

(Section 12 – Melatonin, Alzheimer's disease and Breast Cancer).

The BioInitiative Report of August 31 2007 further states:

"that the evidence from studies on women in the workplace rather strongly suggest that ELF is a risk factor for breast cancer for women with long-term exposures of 10mG and higher". *(Summary for the Public).*

The BioInitiative Report concludes:

"ELF limits for public exposure should be revised to reflect increased risk of breast cancer at environmental levels possibly as low as 2mG or 3mG, certainly as low as 4mG". *(Section 13 – Melatonin – Cell and Animal Studies)*

The Breast Cancer Fund – USA – supports The BioInitiative Report statement that the scientific evidence is sufficient to warrant regulatory action for ELF EMF.

Their recently published *State of the Evidence 2008* available on www.breastcancerfund.org includes information on non-ionising radiation and EMFs.

Breast cancer is the second leading cause of death from cancer in women – second only to lung cancer. As one in every seven women will develop breast cancer in her life it is critical that the public be informed and strategies be implemented that limit ELF EMF exposure in the quest to prevent breast cancer. Lessening the ELF EMF fields we are exposed to – beginning from conception – is recommended.

i   Northrup 2001, p 432
ii   Stevens, Wilson, Anderson in Stevens, Wilson, Anderson, 1997, p.2
iii   Portier 2000, p.1
iv   Cherry 1999, p.11
v   Cherry 1999, p.25
vi   Bushong 2004, p.339
vii   Erren in Stevens, Wilson, Anderson 1997, p.731
viii   Milham 2004, p.86-87

Eleven

Among the most profound environmental consequences of the progression of electrification in societies is: exposure to ELF EMF and light-at-night. ELF EMF (and the variables within it) and light and the roles they play in the disruption of our vital synchronized body rhythms may well help to explain why the risk of developing breast cancer is about five times higher in industrialized nations than it is in underdeveloped countries.

The crucial sleep/wake cycle that sustains our health has changed dramatically with the advent of industrialisation. Artificial dim spectrum-restricted lighting in homes and work situations has replaced dark nights and outside bright, natural full-spectrum lighting during the day. We have changed the natural rhythm of life – work when it is naturally light and sleep when it is naturally dark.

Our bodies are governed by cycles and rhythms that all work in tandem to maintain health and prevent cancer from developing. The rhythms of the various hormones are vital to our health and the role of melatonin in women's lives cannot be underestimated. Melatonin's roles are many: as well as being in present in breast milk melatonin also controls the reproductive cycle.

Dr Joan Borysenko in *A Woman's Life: The Biology, Psychology and Spirituality of the Feminine Life Cycle* states in the days before electric lighting the average age of puberty for girls was fourteen or fifteen. It is now currently between eleven and twelve years of age. With the advent of electric lights our 'days' have become longer which has stimulated the brain's pineal gland to release hormones that bring on puberty several years earlier. Commencing menstruation before 12 years of age is acknowledged as a factor in breast cancer risk.

Further research in the field of body rhythms and cycles is being conducted to provide more answers in the area of breast cancer. "Several studies have strongly suggested that pre-menopausal women who have breast surgery for suspected or already diagnosed breast cancers during the luteal phase of their menstrual cycle have a better prognosis than those who have surgery during another stage of their cycle."[i]   Data has shown that melatonin excretion is highest during the luteal phase of the cycle and lower just prior to ovulation.

It has also been observed that disturbance of body rhythms contribute significantly to the development of breast cancer. "Evidence from observational studies is growing that disturbance of body rhythms in particular, circadian disruption, e.g., shift work or chronic jet-lag contribute significantly to the development of breast cancer".[ii]

Studies on night-shift work and breast cancer risk collectively show an increased breast cancer risk among women. Night-shift work over a long period of time is implicated in breast cancer risk: the longer the time for night-shift work the greater the risk.

The Megdal *et al.*2005 meta-analysis based on thirteen studies (seven of airline cabin crew and six of other night-shift workers) found: "studies on night-shift work and breast cancer risk collectively show an increased breast cancer risk among women".[iii] "Changes in the light-dark exposure (e.g., noonday occupation or trans-meridian travel) shift the timing of the circadian system such that internal rhythms can become desynchronized from both the external environment and internally with each other, impairing our ability to sleep and wake at the appropriate times and compromising physiologic and metabolic processes".[iv]

Flight attendants have a higher risk of breast cancer than those who also partake in night-shift work. (Refer Appendix F). As airline cabin crew pass through areas of differing day length their circadian disruption would be even more affected. This disturbance to the pineal gland, disruption of the melatonin cycle, and the change in the timing of the circadian system reveals how disruption of the pineal gland and melatonin can have severe consequences. As we know that disruption of melatonin is one of the mechanisms involved in the adverse effects of ELF EMF this is supportive of the argument that ELF EMF is a risk factor in breast cancer.

Night-shift work is also a factor for nurses who are also often exposed to the fields from electrical/medical equipment. People who work in areas with high concentrations of electrical equipment are also reported at risk.

Is it possible for ELF EMF exposure to so increase the risk of breast cancer as to produce an excess of cases in a relatively short time period? Epidemiological studies in men lend support for this contention.

Effects in regard to rhythm disturbances in regard to breast cancer risk are proving to be of vital importance with maintaining the integrity of the melatonin signal (e.g., reducing exposure to or ingestion of substances that interfere with the pineal gland and melatonin) seen as paramount. Quality sleep in total darkness preferably at night in a rhythmic pattern is desirable – the use of night-lights while sleeping is discouraged. Sleeping away from electromagnetic fields is recommended. This would include: sleeping away from alarm clocks, electrical equipment and not having electrical equipment and the meter box on the wall behind where you are sleeping. For children this can be critical.

Melatonin has recently been identified as the first anticancer signal to be identified in humans that directly links the central circadian clock with the regulation of human breast cancer development. Blask *et al.* 2005 report: "melatonin is now the first soluble, nocturnal anticancer signal to be identified in humans that directly links the central circadian clock with some of the important mechanisms regulating human breast carcinogenesis and possibly the progression of other malignancies as well".[v]

The field of Chronobiology has identified a multitude of rhythms within our body as well as within each living cell. The circadian rhythm – the most intensively investigated bodily rhythm – is being increasingly recognized as an important tumour suppressor.

The melatonin/serotonin balance is the primary circadian regulator: melatonin and serotonin are the primary circadian hormones. The undisturbed timing of this cycle is crucial for core bodily processes and the cycles that work together and follow each other. The synchronicity of body rhythms is one of the primary roles of the pineal gland and melatonin. Disruption of melatonin is one of the known mechanisms in the adverse affects of ELF EMF. Suppression of the secretion of the hormone melatonin is a precursor to breast cancer. The disturbance/time-shifting of melatonin would subsequently lead to a cascade of hormonal and immune-system changes relevant to the body's cancer-surveillance capacity.

The resetting of the body clock is proving to be important in the treatment (and prevention) of breast cancer as the suprachiasmatic nucleus (SCN) is responsible for controlling circadian rhythms. Research into the effects of ELF EMF and inappropriate and inappropriately-timed artificial light and their interplay must continue in the quest to prevent breast cancer as:

- "Lighting during the night of sufficient intensity can disrupt circadian rhythms, including reduction of circulating melatonin levels and resetting of the circadian pacemaker of the suprachiasmatic nuclei".[vi]

- "Our light quality during the day also appears to affect night-time melatonin production as well as the human circadian pacemaker".[vii]

- "There is evidence that the endogenous melatonin rhythm is stronger for persons in a bright-day environment than in a dim-day environment".[viii]

- "There is evidence "occupational exposure to magnetic fields by day affected the sensitivity of the pineal gland to light exposure that night".[ix]

Moser *et al.* 2006 suggest "that maintenance of a strong circadian rhythm in everyday life and the use of rhythm therapy when disease occurs may not only help to substantially reduce breast cancer incidence and mortality in industrialized countries, but more generally will also support the introduction of new avenues in the prevention and treatment of cancer".[x]

NOTE: The graph in Appendix F showing the different risk factors of breast cancer was provided by Dr Maximilian Moser of the Institute of Noninvasive Diagnosis, Austria. Compiled by Maximilian Moser, Karin Schaumberger, Eva Schernhammer, Richard G Stevens, for the editorial paper *Cancer and Rhythm*, Cancer Causes Control (2006) 17:483–487.

i   Northrup 1998, p.327
ii   Moser *et al.* 2006, p.483
iii   Megdal *et al.* 2005, p.2023-2032
iv   Stevens, 2007 1357-62
v   Blask *et al.* 2005, 65:11174-11184
vi   Stevens 2005, Mar;16(2):254-8
vii   Stevens 2000 at Low frequency EMF, Visible Light, Melatonin and Cancer International Symposium, May 4-5, University of Cologne, Germany
viii   Stevens 2000, p.1
ix   Juutilainen and Kumlin in Henshaw and O'Carroll 2007, point 6
x   Moser *et al.* 2006, p.486

Twelve

*E*ven though the ELF EMF and breast cancer scientific debate has been the subject of continued controversy for over two decades breast cancer has been the only cancer for which there has been a plausible and specific biological mechanism proposed from quite early on.

The 'Melatonin Hypothesis', theorized by Dr Richard Stevens in 1987 was based on the assumption that magnetic field exposure affects melatonin production in the same way as light-at-night and that melatonin is protective against breast cancer, possibly by affecting the level of oestrogen. (Low circulating melatonin may be related directly to risk of breast cancer, or may be related through its impact on oestrogen, or both; reduced melatonin levels increase the level of circulating oestrogen, which would increase susceptibility to sex hormone-related cancers).

The Melatonin Hypothesis

The 'Melatonin Hypothesis' is:

> exposure to 'light at night' and/or EMF may disrupt the function of the pineal gland and its primary hormone melatonin, and that this disruption lowers melatonin production, a consequence that may lead to an increase in the long-term risk of breast cancer. [i]

At the time when the 'Melatonin Hypothesis' was presented it was not known whether ELF EMF affected pineal melatonin production in experimental animals and/or humans. There was also no experimental evidence for increased breast cancer development or growth in response to ELF EMF exposure.

Shortly after Loscher and colleagues substantiated the melatonin hypothesis by carrying out a series of experiments designed expressly to test the 'Melatonin Hypothesis' in female rats. "Collectively, the data demonstrated that long-term ELF EMF exposure of female rats (DMBA – treated) promotes the growth of mammary tumours in a highly dose-related fashion, thus substantiating the melatonin hypothesis". [ii]

The 'Melatonin Hypothesis' is based principally on three lines of evidence:

1. Light effects on melatonin production

2. EMF effects on melatonin production

3. The role of melatonin in breast cancer etiology. [iii]

Light Effects on Melatonin

Melatonin suppression by 'light-at-night' is an established fact. Acute exposure to 'light-at-night', if of sufficient intensity, suppresses melatonin production. Even low light intensities can reduce circulating levels of melatonin in humans – the brighter the light the greater the reduction on circulating melatonin. Exposure to 'light-at-night' can suppress, delay, or interrupt the nightly synthesis of melatonin, which in turn may influence behaviour, mood, hormone levels or immune function.

"The statistically significant decrease in breast cancer risk by increasing degree of visual impairment suggests a dose-response relationship between visible light and breast cancer risk". [iv]

EMF Effects on Melatonin Production

Laboratory research has shown that melatonin and ELF EMF can play a key role in the development of cancerous tumours. Melatonin has been shown to reduce human breast cancer cell growth.

Can ELF EMF affect melatonin production in humans? This critical question was not only answered in 1993 by Liburdy *et al.*, a threshold was reported between 2-12mG.

Further to this, Liburdy *et al.* 1993 on reporting that melatonin reduces the growth rate of human breast cancer cells (MCF-7) in culture also found that a 12mG 60 Hz magnetic field can block the ability of melatonin to inhibit breast cancer cell growth.

Harland and Liburdy 1996 further observed that "environmental-level 12-mG, 60Hz magnetic fields partially block tamoxifen's cytostatic action, and completely block melatonin's cytostatic action on human breast cells in vitro".[v] This study was replicated (the hallmark for wide acceptance of scientific study results) and confirmed by Blackman *et al.* 1996. Further replication including the studies of Luben *et al.* 1996, Afzal and Liburdy 1996, Ishido *et al.* 2001 and more recently Girgert *et al.* 2005 have resulted in the 12mG effect resting on a firmer foundation.

Also, breast cancer cells treated with melatonin have resumed growing when exposed to ELF EMF.

The Role of Melatonin in Breast Cancer

As far back as 1997, Liburdy and Loscher remarked: "So far, the most abundant data supporting a role for melatonin as an oncostatic hormone is in the realm of breast cancer (Blask 1993; Stevens *et al.* 1992)".[vi] Previous *in vitro* (test tube) and *in vivo* (animal) research supports a protective association between melatonin and breast cancer development.

Even though clinical case-control studies of melatonin levels in cancer patients and controls display a general association with lower melatonin levels in cancer patients, the debate has centred on whether the cancer itself or the therapy for these cancers is wholly or partly responsible for an association – whether the disease created low melatonin levels or is the disease caused by low melatonin levels.

Most previous studies of the association between circulating melatonin levels and breast cancer risk in humans are limited because melatonin levels were measured after the subjects were diagnosed with breast cancer. Schernhammer & Hankinson (2005) is a more recent **prospective** study showing that higher melatonin levels (as measured in first morning urine) are associated with a lower risk of breast cancer.

The testing of melatonin levels and urine concentration of melatonin has been conducted in many studies yet of paramount importance is also the suppressed function/changed behaviour of melatonin and what the effects are downstream. "The mechanisms underlying the direct anti-proliferative effect of melatonin in the mammary gland involve a melatonin receptor-mediated down-regulation of estrogen receptors, increased expression of the tumour suppressor gene p53, a reduction of DNA synthesis, and effects on calcium homeostasis".[vii] In 2001, Masami Ishido at Japan's National Institute for Environmental Studies found that the magnetic field disrupts the cells' signalling system – their internal communications network – which determines how they respond to their environment.

The validating work of Dr David Blask and colleagues also features in melatonin/ELF EMF breast cancer research and more recently, the very important Blask *et al.* 2005 paper is an explicit demonstration that the normal concentration of melatonin in human blood *per se* suppresses human breast cancer growth. Blood was taken from women sleeping at night containing the normal concentration of melatonin. They fed it to rats that had human breast tumours transplanted into them. The blood effectively halted the growth of these tumours in the rats. Blood collected during the day or after a white light exposure during the night did not.

Oestrogen dominance plays a role in breast cancer with melatonin playing a vital role in breast cancer protection· when melatonin levels are low oestrogen levels are high. High levels of oestrogen stimulate oestrogen-sensitive breast cancer. Melatonin competes with oestrogens for the existing receptor sites. More recent research indicates "night-time melatonin is a relevant anti-cancer signal to human breast cancers. Ninety percent of human breast cancers have specific receptors for this signal."[viii]

Further Investigation

Like the pineal gland the pituitary gland is also part of the endocrine system dependent on circadian homeostasis, secreting hormones regulating homeostasis and controlling the secretion of hormones by other endocrine glands. At puberty, the pineal gland switches on the reproductive hormones of the pituitary and the pituitary in turn, activates the ovaries which start making oestrogen and progesterone.

An investigation of a cluster of so-called 'brain' tumors associated with ELF EMF in a case-control study showed that some of the tumors were in fact malignancies of the pituitary gland. (Floderus *et al.* 1993).

Dr Thomas C Erren MPH, of the Institute and Policlinic for Occupational and Social Medicine, University of Cologne, Germany stated: "If a malignant transition of the pituitary gland is confirmed in subsequent studies, this would support the concept of a hormone-mediated pathway between ELF EMF and cancer".[ix]

Dr Erren also commented: "recent epidemiologic findings of excessive breast cancer cases and tumors of the pituitary gland in Swedish railway workers are consistent with the general notion that ELF EMF may affect inter-related hormone-dependent organs (Floderus *et al.* 1994)".[x]

Refer to Appendix G for the hypothetical graph (updated by Dr Erren in 1997) on how breast cancer could develop from ELF EMF exposure.

The Breast Cancer ELF EMF Dilemma

The ELF EMF breast cancer link in women has been a hotly debated topic since first proposed. As it seriously questions how we as a society conduct our daily lives the mere premise continues to be questioned.

In the more recent Forss'en *et al.* 2005 study *Occupational Magnetic Fields and Female Breast Cancer: A Case-Control Study using Swedish Population Registers and New Exposure Data* – one of the largest studies ever on occupational electromagnetic field exposure and breast cancer risk – the authors found "no evidence for an increased risk of breast cancer among women working in occupations with high magnetic field exposure".[xi] The authors concluded "the findings give no support to the hypothesis that magnetic field exposure increases the risk of female breast cancer".[xii]

Following the Forss'en *et al.* study the Feychting and Forssen paper 2006 *Electromagnetic fields and female breast cancer* was released. This paper relied heavily on the Forssen *et al.* 2005 study referred to above and concluded: "…one must conclude that the weight of the evidence available today suggests that power frequency magnetic field exposure most likely is not a risk factor for breast cancer development".[xiii]

The widely disseminated Forss'en *et al.* study may enable decision makers and those with vested interests to ignore the ELF EMF breast cancer link in women.

Also, very carefully conducted studies of residential wire codes and in-home measurements have not seen associations. These studies are not proof of no effect, but also do not support a strong effect of ELF EMF and breast cancer.

From the data accessed to date in regard to the 'Melatonin Hypothesis' the case for light is looking 'possibly' strong and the case for ELF EMF weak due to mixed evidence in the studies and being considerably weakened with the Forss'en *et al.* study and Feytching and Forss'en paper. Exposure to light-at-night or EMF can decrease production of melatonin by the pineal gland. Of the two, "light inhibits melatonin much more strongly and more reproducibly than magnetic fields may".[xiv] Much of the effect though, but probably not all, is dependent on melatonin.

Yet The BioInitiative Report of 2007 comments that the Forss'en *et al.* 2005 study may be considered influential, unless reviewed in detail. The BioInitiative Report provides detailed information regarding the exposure misclassification.
(*Section 12 – Evidence For Effects On Melatonin: Alzheimer's Disease and Breast Cancer – Section IV.E. – Occupational Case-Control Studies of MF Exposure as a Risk Factor for Breast Cancer* – Points 41-44 – Zoreh Davanipour, DVM, PhD Eugene Sobel, PhD).

Also, Dr Erren in *Letters to the Editor* (Am J Epidemiol 2005;162:389–395) comments that in studies of possible links between non-ionising radiation and breast cancer, exposure misclassification is of paramount concern. Feychting and Forss'en comment that "exposure misclassification is still a concern in studies of magnetic field exposure and cancer risk, especially since it is unknown which aspect of the exposure would be biologically relevant, should an effect exist".[xv]

Estimating exposure conditions can never compare to the actual exposure conditions (and the myriad of ELF EMF variables) that present in real cases of breast cancer, excessive breast cancer cases and breast cancer clusters that are ELF EMF related.

The Masking of ELF EMF

It is the comments by Dr Thomas Erren on the latest Feytching and Forss'en 2006 paper in *Letters to the Editor* (Am J Epidemiol 2005;162:389–395) that may hold the key to the answers we seek.

Dr Erren discusses confounding (in which a measure of the effect of an intervention or exposure is distorted because of the association of exposure with other factor(s) that influence the outcome under study) with light in the Forss'en *et al.* study.

Dr Erren further comments:

> ...since the possibly strong risk factor light was not controlled for, **it remains conceivable that magnetic fields do increase breast cancer risks but that this effect has been assessed erroneously in many (or all) epidemiologic studies to date**.

> Possibly, the control of light (indeed, all animals were exposed to the same light regime) **may have allowed the experimental researchers to detect magnetic field effects that could be masked** in the existing epidemiologic studies by uncontrolled light exposures. [xvi]

Artificial light and ELF EMF are both non-ionising radiation. Light and the fact that we are all exposed to ELF EMF can contribute to masking the ELF EMF effect in the development of breast cancer.

i   Stevens, Wilson, Anderson in Stevens, Wilson, Anderson, 1997, p.2
ii   Loscher, 2000 at Low frequency EMF, Visible Light, Melatonin and Cancer International Symposium, May 4-5 2000, University of Cologne, Germany
iii Stevens, Wilson, Anderson in Stevens, Wilson, Anderson, 1997, p.741
iv Verkasalo *et al.* 2000 at Low frequency EMF, Visible Light, Melatonin and Cancer International Symposium, May 4-5 2000, University of Cologne, Germany
v   Liburdy and Harland in Stevens, Wilson, Anderson 1997, p.689
vi Liburdy and Loscher in Stevens, Wilson, Anderson 1997, p.643
vii Fedrowitz, Kamino, Loscher 2004, p.249
viii Blask at American Association for Cancer Research 2003
ix Erren in Stevens, Wilson, Anderson 1997, p.705
x   Erren in Stevens, Wilson, Anderson 1997, p.705
xi Forss'en *et al.* 2005, p.255
xii Forss'en *et al.* 2005, p.258
xiii Feychting and Forss'en 2006, p.557
xiv Erren in Letters to the Editor, p.392
xv Feychting and Forss'en 2006, p.557
xvi Erren 2005, p.392-393

Thirteen

*T*he question behind all the research in regard to the ELF EMF enigma is how these fields create disease.

EMF is being associated with increased disease states which leaves unresolved the exact mechanism(s) that are involved. Did exposure to these fields directly cause cancer or did exposure to these fields cause reactions in the body that allowed cancer to develop?

Dr Cherry had travelled extensively, talking to original researchers, collating research data and hypothesized how serious disease and cancer could result from ELF EMF exposure. In the US he also visited the Environmental Protection Agency (EPA) talking to scientists researching EMF and biological effects.

One of the most important signals in our bodies – calcium ions – operates in the vicinity of 50 Hz frequency. The frequency of ELF EMF by coincidence is 50 Hz. Is it possible that one of the most important signals in our bodies and ELF EMF are interacting at a core level? Both are extremely low frequency oscillating electromagnetic signals. One is natural and fundamental to life, the other is man-made and artificial.

The calcium ion frequency is mathematical fact. Mathematics is often way ahead of what science can establish as valid.

How Our Bodies Could Detect These Fields

To explain how our bodies might detect these fields an example is when an opera singer achieves a certain note and a glass shatters. This is called 'resonance' – magnetic resonance – because the frequencies match.

In the medical field today *Magnetic Resonance Imaging* (MRI) is used to allow physicians to better evaluate parts of the body and certain diseases that may not be assessed adequately with other imaging methods such as x-ray, ultrasound or CT scans. MRI uses a powerful rapidly changing magnetic field, radio waves and a computer to produce detailed pictures of organs, soft tissues, bone and virtually all other internal body structures. (MRI use is increasing as it does not use ionising radiation – x-rays). The MRI signal 'tunes' to the body.

Professor Ross Adey followed by Carl Blackman PhD and colleagues reported that the biophysical mechanism for detecting and responding to external ELF signals, resulting in reduced melatonin, occurs through resonant absorption of the ELF signals in the brain. Dr Cherry's theoretical model also incorporated resonance absorption as a way for weak fields to have a biological influence. The entire resonance theory "provides logical mechanisms whereby single cells and specific organs such as the pineal gland may intercept and derive information from electromagnetic fields".[ii]

There is a natural magnetic field in the atmosphere, which tends to oscillate at very low frequencies and it is these oscillations that were first detected by Schumann and Konig in 1954. (The generation, transmission, and use of electric energy are associated with the production of weak electric and magnetic fields which oscillate 50 or 60 times/second). The discovery of the Schumann Resonances, predicted by German physicist W. O. Schumann between 1952 and 1957, indicates that the Earth behaves like an enormous electric circuit. The Schumann Resonances – quasi-standing electromagnetic waves that exist in the Earth's electromagnetic cavity – are the natural and vital orchestrating pulse for life on our planet. These pulses travel many times per second completely around the world between our planet's surface and the ionosphere, sending co-ordinating signals to all organisms that connect us to the global electrostatic field.

Dr Cherry maintained there is strong evidence that the Schumann Resonances (a timing signal which is absorbed through resonance and detected and responded to by the brain) continually provide an external synchronisation signal to assist all mammals to maintain their brain, heart and cellular timing homeostasis. "German research has proven that human brains detect and use the Schumann Resonances (SR) for timing synchronization".[iii] Dr Cherry suggested that there could be a causal link between melatonin and the Schumann Resonances as this natural ELF signal that propagates around the world with a diurnal and seasonal pattern follows the human diurnal melatonin pattern. (The Northern California Earthquake Data Center computes and archives

Schumann Resonance data).

If the human brain is dependant on being tuned into the natural low frequency ELF signal of the Schumann Resonances (SR) would it follow that any interference to this process would surely disturb this life-supporting process? Is it possible that the man-made artificial low frequency ELF signal interfers with the crucial homeostasis of the earth's natural low frequency ELF signal (SR) and the natural internal low frequency ELF fields that keeps our systems functioning properly minimising the risk of serious disease and cancer?

Melatonin

Melatonin has been shown to play a vital role in protecting our systems from contracting cancer. Disruption of the natural production of melatonin is one of the mechanisms involved in the adverse health effects attributed to ELF EMF.

It has been established that the cycle of the day's sunshine and the darkness of night affect the timing of the body's manufacture of the hormone melatonin. It has also been reported that production of the biological timing hormone, melatonin, can be affected by magnetic fields.

Melatonin, released by the pineal gland in darkness, is the most potent natural antioxidant known that is vital for regulating the crucial daily circadian (nearly 24 hour resulting from the variation of light during the day) rhythm.

One of the main functions of the pineal gland is the release of melatonin. Melatonin production which can influence behaviour, mood, hormone levels and immune function is 50-70 times greater at night during sleep, triggered by a signal from the eye indicating that light is falling below a certain threshold, sensing the absence of light.

Melatonin, which enhances the effectiveness of the immune system, is carried by the circulation system throughout the body passing through the cell membrane, scavenging the highly toxic free radicals in the cell to protect the DNA in every cell. The work of Professor Russel Reiter – prominent in the field of melatonin and melatonin/ELF EMF – has reported that while the Blood Brain Barrier (BBB) denies access to most free radical scavengers, melatonin has free access and that melatonin's ability to enter every cell is important for melatonin's function as an antioxidant.

Disruption of melatonin disturbs our internal rhythmic processes leading to a cascade of events that compromises our body's defense systems which can lead to cancer.

It is reported that blind and partially sighted people – whose melatonin levels are increased because of the missing light effect – have lower breast cancer rates than sighted people. What is the connection? More research is being conducted in this area. Melatonin is the primary vehicle by which light information is translated into a biological signal. If melatonin is affected by magnetic fields, do magnetic fields give the impression that light is present all the time, therefore affecting melatonin's cancer suppressing role? If magnetic fields induce currents in the brain or in the pineal gland how would this occur?

The Magnetic Field of the Earth

All living organisms are exposed to naturally produced electromagnetic fields/radiation generated by the earth, the sun, and the rest of the cosmos.

The earth has a steady magnetic field that forms the basis for navigation – earth's magnetic field causes a compass needle to orient in a North-South direction. In the 1960s Dr Robert Becker and Dr Howard Friedman found "a significant relationship between the rate of admissions for people with schizophrenia and manic-depressive psychosis and the occurrence of major magnetic storms".[i] There is now very extensive and well established literature (previously unconsidered in the EMF field) that animals across a wide range of species detect tiny changes in the Earth's magnetic field for the purposes of navigation.

(Refer Wiltschko & Wiltschko 2006 *Magnetoreception BioEssays* 28. 157-168).

Calcium Ions

Our neurochemistry is subject to delicate processes governed by natural ELF signals. Each cell has an encoder and receiver to transmit, receive and respond to messages, which form an amazing biological communication network. Professor Adey – one of the most respected EMF veterans – referred to this as the cells 'whispering' to each other.

Our sight, thoughts, memories, learning and emotions use complex oscillating electromagnetic signals. We are electromagnetically sensitive beings and the brain is electrically and magnetically sensitive. The brain – as well as various muscles – has electrical activity that produces internal electric fields throughout the body. The heart is also an electromagnetic organ with an electric pulse that initiates a cascade of calcium ions that causes the cells in the heart to contract and produce a heartbeat. The electrocardiogram, magnetocardiogram, electroencephalograph and magneto-encephalograph are used to measure the electric and magnetic fields in the body for diagnostic purposes.

As the language of the brain is electrical it is the most electrically sensitive organ in our body. The brain is a massive source of ELF signals that get transmitted throughout the body allowing messages to flow through the central nervous system (CNS). The CNS provides a cable system to carry electrical signals to body organs.

The brain and nervous system operate using highly complex patterns of electrical signals. Our cells use oscillating ELF signals for many vital functions. One of the most vital communication signalling processes is the calcium ion signalling process.

The brain communicates with the organs and the cells of the body using enzymes, hormones and ion currents. The chemical link between EMF and life processes is believed to be ions, especially calcium ions as it has been shown that external EMF clearly affects the electrical properties and ion distribution around cells. Virtually all of the physiological/biological processes in our bodies involve ions. The calcium ion is one of the most important substances in cells.

Calcium functions as a vital intercellular and intracellular messenger. Disruption of this vital process leads to other biochemical events and physiological changes: accelerated cell proliferation rate, chromosomal damage, cell stress and immune system impairment which reduces the body's cancer surveillance capacity and ability to kill transformed cells. The alteration of the vital cellular calcium ion concentrations is a well-established biological effect from many independent laboratories, particularly from the work of Professor Adey (Bawin & Adey) and Carl Blackman.

Just as melatonin is the bio-chemical signal for darkness, living cells are bio-electric-chemical structures – every cell in our body has low frequency energy. Every cell in our bodies utilises calcium – it is fundamental to the processes that keep us alive. Calcium ions as mediators of intracellular signalling are crucial for apoptosis – programmed cell death that removes damaged cells. Reduced apoptosis leads to an accumulation of faulty cells.

Professor Adey explained in his correspondence to our group that the model of calcium-ELF field interaction is known as a "cyclotron resonance model", which was first proposed by Carl Blackman PhD at the Environmental Protection Agency and substantially extended by Dr Abraham Liboff at Oakland University in Michigan in a series of papers from the late 1980s to the mid 1990s. Dr Liboff developed and published experiments showing biological responses that were consistent with predicted calcium ion resonances.

Dr Cherry hypothesized that external ELF signals induce alterations in the calcium ion signals that in turn send signals to the pineal gland that alters the melatonin/serotonin balance. This is transferred to the body organs through the Central Nervous System (CNS) and hormone/enzyme/ion cellular signalling system.

ELF EMF

is detected by the brain

which alters the cellular ion concentration	which reduces pineal melatonin production
which allows more damaged cells to survive	which allows more free radicals to damage cells
reducing the competence of the immune system	reducing the competence of the immune system

INCREASES CANCER RISK

The ELF signal systems within cells also involve calcium ions that can be directly interfered with by external ELF signals.

Dr Cherry contended that ELF modulated EMF reduces melatonin and alters the calcium ion homeostasis in cells, supported by multiple independent studies showing that 50/60 Hz fields damage chromosomes, break DNA strands and impair immune system competence.

Cells with damaged DNA either die or the DNA is repaired. If repaired correctly there are no further problems. DNA that is not entirely repaired or not repaired correctly leads to changes in chromosomes and mutations that can lead to the development of cancer. DNA damage and altered cell function can accelerate tumour development. "Critical genetic mutations in one single cell are sufficient to lead to cancer".[iv] Damage to the genetic information within the cell (DNA) can increase the risk of cancer, neurological, cardiac and reproductive damage, illness and death. DNA stability is vital for the prevention of defects in further generations.

It is becoming increasingly clear that we are governed by internal body rhythms and cycles and their synchronization is proving vital in the defense against serious disease and cancer. Each chemical has its own cycle of highs and lows, interacting with and influencing the other cycles. Any disruption in the timing of our bodily systems has the ability to prevent the cancer surveillance capacity operating at its optimal level, therefore compromising the immune system.

Dr Cherry maintained that substances that reduce melatonin are genotoxic because of the reduced antioxidant effect allowing the highly toxic free radicals to cause more genetic damage. If melatonin is reduced the natural ability of the body to fight cancerous cells can be compromised resulting in a more aggressive spread of cancer.

Cancer is characterised by cell division that has gone out of control. Like all cancers, breast cancer develops over a period of time arising when there is an imbalance between breast tissue cell growth and breast tissue cell death: excessive and uncontrolled cell division, and a lack of normal, healthy programmed cell death. These fields seem to promote cancer by changes in the rate at which cells divide and differentiate. Calcium ions as mediators of intracellular signalling are crucial for apoptosis – programmed cell death that removes damaged cells. Breast cancer also depends on the ability of the pineal gland to properly secrete melatonin, which assists in regulating cell division and multiplication.

Dr Cherry maintained: "External ELF signals induce alterations in the calcium ion signals that in turn send signals to the pineal gland that alters the melatonin/serotonin balance".

<hr>

As calcium ions perform many functions in cells and tissues more testing of specific signalling pathways is needed to identify which biological process is affected by the calcium change. It has not been unequivocally demonstrated that ELF EMF can lower melatonin in humans: observational studies in humans have shown associations of exposure with lower levels of melatonin whereas the short term laboratory experiments in humans are negative.

Further research is still being conducted to reveal the exact processes involved to further explain: the adverse effects and if the Cherry hypothesis is valid.

i   Becker 1990, p.89
ii   Becker 1990, p.238
iii Cherry 1999, p.1
iv   Lai 2007, point 5

Fourteen

*E*ven though this book has concentrated mainly on high magnetic fields an additional culprit is emerging: high frequency voltage transients – transient electromagnetic fields. Most of the research on the biological effects of non-ionising radiation has looked at one of two frequency ranges: 50/60 Hz (ELF EMF) and 800 MHz to 2.5 GHz (RF EMF). 'Dirty Electricity' which flows along and radiates from wires involves both ELF EMF and RF EMF. Having characteristics of ELF EMF and RF EMF it lies in an intermediate frequency range (at the low end of the RF spectrum). Results are strongly suggesting that transients are biologically active and at intensities currently found in homes and schools.

The study of Dr Samuel Milham and Lloyd Morgan of the teacher's cancer cluster at La Quinta Middle School, USA, provides critical insights into the importance of an electrically clean environment. They concluded that: "the cancer incidence in the teachers at this school was unusually high and is strongly associated with high frequency voltage transients, which may be a universal carcinogen, similar to ionizing radiation".

(Refer Milham, S MD MPH, Morgan LL BS, 2008 *A new electromagnetic exposure metric: high frequency voltage transients associated with increased cancer incidence in teachers in a California school*, AM J Ind Med, May 29; 51: (8) 579-586.)

Samuel Milham MD MPH – retired Washington State Department of Health – a leading epidemiologist and recipient of the prestigious Ramazzini Award (1997) was the first to link workers exposed to EMFs with higher rates of leukemia in 1982. L Lloyd Morgan BS is a retired electronics engineer and has been Director of the Central Brain Tumour Registry of the United States (CBTRUS).

Since the introduction of electricity and the rapid growth in our use of electronic devices the quality of electrical power flowing along wires within homes, schools and workplaces has been deteriorating. 'Dirty electricity', also known as 'dirty power', has increased dramatically since the late 1970s with increasing intensity. With the advent of computers in the 1980s that periodically 'malfunctioned' more prominent attention has been bought to 'dirty electricity'.

'Dirty electricity' includes: poor power quality, incorrect wiring and the transients and spikes created from turning equipment and switches on and off resulting in RF EMF which can travel along electrical wires. Transients can pack a big burst of energy into a short period of time and are a type of unwanted modulation that are caused by motors, switches and electrical devices being switched on and off throughout the power grid. A spike is a type of transient. These spikes and transients are effectively a high-frequency signal that is now superimposed on the original sine wave. When produced, 'dirty electricity' can also enter other work stations/buildings/households that share transformers. Generated outside the building it enters the building on electric wiring and through ground rod and conductive plumbing.

Electromagnetic pollution in the form of 'dirty electricity', ground current, and radio frequency radiation from wireless devices is also increasing at an alarming rate. 'Dirty electricity' is a global problem with the suggestion that it can be a contributing factor in many health disorders that have also been increasing at an alarming rate, including: asthma, ADD/ADHD, multiple sclerosis, chronic fatigue, and fibromyalgia.

The studies of Magda Havas – Associate Professor Environmental & Resource Studies, Trent University, Ontario, Canada and Dave Stetzer – President of Stetzer Electric in Wisconsin – suggest 'dirty electricity' may be:

- interfering with education in schools and possibly contributing to disruptive behaviour associated with attention deficit disorder (ADD)

- exacerbating symptoms for those suffering from tinnitus and multiple sclerosis

- contributing to electrical hypersensitivity

More studies are being conducted to research the interplay between electromagnetic pollution and these disorders.

Diabetes

In addition to lifestyle and genetics, the environment appears to be another factor contributing to high levels of blood sugar. Doctors have long suspected an environmental component but it has not been until now that one has been found. Dr Magda Havas has just labeled environmental diabetes as Type 3 diabetes. Type 3 refers to a diabetic whose blood sugar is also affected by an environmental trigger - 'dirty electricity' increases blood sugar in Type 3 diabetics. 'Dirty electricity' is one such trigger and other triggers are also suspected. By closely following plasma glucose levels in four Type 1 and Type 2 diabetics, Dr Havas found that they responded directly to the amount of 'dirty electricity' in their environment. In an electromagnetically clean environment:

- Type 1 diabetics have been shown to require less insulin; and

- Type 2 diabetics have been shown to have lower levels of plasma glucose.

Dr Havas and David Stetzer have worked with individuals who have both Type 1 and Type 2 diabetes and those who are pre-diabetic and have found that blood sugar levels can change rapidly (within a matter of 20 minutes or so for some individuals) as they move from an environment that is electrically dirty to one that is electrically clean (and back again). Dr Havas suggests that 'dirty electricity' may explain why brittle diabetics have difficulty regulating blood sugar. Exercise on a treadmill, which produces 'dirty electricity' has been shown to increase plasma glucose.

Dr Havas reports exposure to electromagnetic pollution in its various forms may account for higher plasma glucose levels and may contribute to the misdiagnosis of diabetes. It is suggested that diagnosis of diabetes needs to be done in an electromagnetically clean environment to prevent misdiagnosis and to properly assess the severity of this disorder. Most medical centers have electronic equipment and use fluorescent lights that produce 'dirty electricity', which is likely to cause abnormally high blood sugar readings for those with a combination of diabetes and electrohypersensitivity (Type 3 diabetes). It is reported that the results from case studies have been so dramatic further investigation is warranted.

Dr Havas comments that based on estimates of people who suffer from symptoms of electrical hypersensitivity (3–35%), as many as 5–60 million diabetics worldwide may be affected.

A newer exposure metric

The fast-paced growth in technology has introduced further interactions. Mobile or broadcast antennas (RF EMF/MW) can also contribute to high frequencies on electrical wires in nearby buildings. High voltage powerlines can also emit radio frequency fields. RF signals of cell phones often are modulated at ELF. Power supplies, light sources, computers and other electric devices can radiate RF through coil systems that are used to produce magnetic and ELF EMF stimuli. The work of Adey (1990) and other scientists has shown that ELF-modulated RF EMF can be a very potent biological stimulus.

As a consequence of poor power quality surge suppressors are commonly used to protect sensitive electronic equipment. Industry uses large capacitors to protect sensitive equipment from power surges and now filters are being used to alleviate the symptoms of many health disorders.

Martin Graham, an Emeritus Professor of Electrical Engineering at the University of California, Berkeley and power quality expert, Dave Stetzer, have designed a filter that can be used inside buildings to clean the power that enters the building as well as the 'dirty electricity' generated within the building. 'Dirty electricity' can now be monitored with measuring equipment (microsurge meters) and reduced with filters (Graham/Stetzer filters) that are providing valuable information for research into this newer field.

Presented at the World Health Organization Workshop of Electrical Hypersensitivity in 2004 Dr Havas and Dave Stetzer produced studies showing that symptoms of electrohypersensitivity are reduced with GS filters. Individuals diagnosed with multiple sclerosis have reported better balance and fewer tremors. Those requiring a cane walked unassisted within a few days to weeks after GS filters were installed in their home. The filters are now also available for in-home use.

Further information and details of Graham/Stetzer filters and the Stetzerizer™ meter are available at:

www.stetzerelectric.com

Fifteen

*W*hile the birth of the new day is gradual almost melancholy in tropical Queensland where I am lucky enough to live, the night comes ever so swiftly with definite abruptness as the light is extinguished. Further north in the lush rainforests and in coastal beaches night time is the time to immerse one's senses in a walk along a beach to see the moon beams gently waltzing across the waves at full moon and to listen to the waves hissing serpent-like on the ghostly whitened sand. The heavy banging of the waves against the rocks often reminds me of the knocks of life and of late, the knocks I've had to absorb on the campaign trail in my effort to take on the authorities and convince them to clean electricity by 2020 – or sooner would be all the better.

As I come from pioneering stock I often think how tough it was for pioneers in Australia to build a nation on their long journey. For me this comparatively minor journey of "hard rock and soft water" has been dramatic. The pioneers' struggle reminds me in a minor way how hard it was for the early pioneers to convince authorities, sitting on their thoroughbreds, to listen to their ideas and to get some positive changes in their everyday life. Australia's favourite son and troubadour, Banjo Paterson who wrote the words of "Waltzing Matilda" comes to mind. All of us know that we can't sing "Waltzing Matilda" without visualizing the brown faces under wide-brimmed Diggers hats, of Tobruk "Rats" – the real spirit of Australia.

In Australia there has been present from the earliest days a spunky spirit of "can do" and I'm pleased to say that I have inherited such a trait from my pioneering ancestors. Men and often women in those days pushed hard from the coast in tilted wagons and bullock drays and families that were scattered met and swapped experiences and gave opinions often verbose and urgent but always sincere in shearing sheds and around secure campfires. They got together not only to swap stories but discuss definite improvements to their "lot"......to make things better for not just the individual but for all and sundry. They listened, they questioned while they searched for a better way to live and in so doing they fought to win a true democracy. These were tough people who spotted a "bull-duster" a mile away and sensed authenticity and were irreverent towards pompous, arrogant, unimaginative officialdom. Similarly, now in my work for achieving clean electricity I've met the pompous, the arrogant in business and government who put profit and power before the people. These are the people I have had to face who are hell-bent on denying justice to groups such as ours and who continue to deny that "dirty" electricity is a threat to the health and well-being of people. These are also people who in my opinion practice the highest form of self-deception and in so doing put people – thousands upon thousands – at risk. During the Energex court case I met a great number of such individuals and it shocked me. I realise I was naïve but frankly the attitude of some of the so-called high officials and learned people was bordering on misogyny and paternalism and definitely patronizing as I was treated as the "little woman" who had come out of the kitchen, who should go back and why was she ever allowed out in the first place? What got me through was not only my determination and the inspiration I had gained from my leadership teaching in Western Australia but also the good sense of humour of those around me coupled to a good notion of social justice and that great Australian ability to turn a severe matter into a yarn to securely impress one another to keep moving forward.

For all environmentalists today I say this is our time for change. Together and intelligently we can clean the planet.

I am for one up for the challenge and as I look ahead I see my walk will be filled with adventure, surprises and victories as now I have been joined by even a bigger collection of highly skilled, capable and dynamic people who like me carry the early bush spirit of "can do". What's important is that they are convinced not by me only but also by the body of evidence that proves that "dirty" electricity can kill and has more than just a tenuous link to breast cancer and other diseases.

This talented group and myself intend leading a campaign to clean up electricity and will be doing it through creating greater awareness, making accessible the evidence to prove the case and then to seek appropriate legislation in the parliament to regulate electricity so that it can be safe for us and future generations. The first step is awareness of what is happening in the officialdom ranks as they scramble for a cover-up, hence this book and any subsequent book that will make more and more evidence available for all to see.

Deep into the night in Queensland when I burn the midnight oil, I can hear the sounds of the night……. the extraordinary sound of the catbird at first, followed by the symphony giving way to the dawn chorus as the cycle begins again and that is what my campaign and campaigns for clean energy will follow, day in and day out until we achieve **CLEAN ELECTRICITY FOR AUSTRALIA** – once more the sooner this happens the better for all of us not only for Australia but worldwide.

Not only am I inspired by the wildlife symphony in the dawn and dusk I am too motivated by the inspirational human voices especially those of the late great Pavarotti and Sarah Brightman when performing "Nessun Dorma" None Shall Sleep…….so beautiful and directional for me and that's the promise I've made to myself, my family, my friends and for those Aussies who care – until the mission is accomplished there will be no rest!

Nessun Dorma

Want more information on the 'Donna Fisher Silent Fields Inc.'?

Want to help? Want to join the campaign?

Visit our website: silentfields.com

or

Contact: donnafisher@silentfields.com

Glossary

Acute effects	effects caused by being in a high field for a short time.
Aetiological	cause or origin.
ALARA	As Low As Reasonably Achievable, economic and social factors being taken into account.
ALL	Acute Lymphoblastic (lymphoid) Leukaemia.
ALS	Amyotrophic Lateral Sclerosis, the most common form of Motor Neurone Disease.
AML	Acute Myeloid Leukaemia.
Antioxidant	compounds that metabolise the dangerous free radicals.
Biophysics	a scientific discipline for understanding how the natural body's electromagnetic and biological systems work.
Blood-Brain Barrier	a membrane that goes right around the brain protecting it from unwanted chemicals in the blood stream.
Cancer cluster	a greater than expected number of cases of a particular disease, with a group of people, a geographical area, or a period of time.
Calcium ion efflux	leads to the survival of damaged cells which carry their chromosome aberrations into future generations of cells.
Cell proliferation	the act of a single cell or group of cells reproducing and multiplying in number.
Confounding	a situation in which a measure of the effect of an intervention or exposure is distorted because of the association of exposure with other factor(s) that influence the outcome under study.
Cytostatic	Inhibiting or suppressing cellular growth and multiplication.
DMBA	a chemical carcinogen – 7,12-dimethylbenz(a)anthracene.
DNA	is a nucleic acid molecule that contains the genetic instructions used in the development and functioning of all living things. Our genetic code of life. How we reproduce and replicate cells.
Dose	the amount of an agent that reaches a particular target organ over a specified period of time.
Dose-response	the relationship between the dose and the effect it produces.
EFs	electric fields.
ELF	extremely low frequency (often termed extra low frequency). The newer term, weak low intensity EMF is also being used.
ELF EMF	covers the frequency range of 3Hz to 300Hz.
EMF	electric, magnetic and electromagnetic fields. Are associated with electricity, whether it be from manufactured sources such as power generation or from natural processes going on within animal or plant cells.

EME	electromagnetic energy (often used for EMF/EMR).
EMR	electromagnetic radiation
Endogenous	made by the body or brain.
Epidemiology	the study of the various factors influencing the occurrence, distribution, prevention, and control of disease, injury, and other health-related events in a defined human population. Epidemiological studies imply the analysis of a statistical connection between exposure and disease. A statistical connection does not mean that the exposure causes the disease.
Oestrogen	a hormone produced primarily by the ovaries and testes. Important for the maintenance of normal brain function and development of nerve cells.
Free radicals	unstable molecules, produced naturally by the body, which, if not neutralized by antioxidants, can damage or destroy cell's structures and DNA. In excess they are thought to be one of the main culprits responsible for many disease processes, including Alzheimer's disease, Parkinson's disease, MS, heart disease, cancer. Antioxidants help minimize free-radical damage.
Frequency	the number of complete cycles of an electromagnetic wave in a second. Unit: hertz, abbreviation: Hz. 1 Hz = 1 cycle per second.
FSH	follicle stimulating hormone.
Gamma ray	emitted after nuclear reactions, shares the high-frequency end of the electromagnetic spectrum with x-rays, which have similar properties.
Gauss	a common unit of measurement of AC magnetic field strength. Tesla is also used.
Gauss meter	an instrument that measures the strength of AC magnetic fields.
Gene p53	regulates the cell cycle, helps to suppress cancer. p53 has been described as "the guardian of the genome", and the "master watchman", referring to its role in preventing genome mutation.
Genotoxic	any evidence of genetic damage, cell death or neoplastic transformation. Any substance that damages DNA or chromosomes. A genotoxic substance is mutagenic, carcinogenic and teratogenic. Genotoxic substances can cause cancer, reproductive health effects and neurological damage.
Grounding	electricity returns to earth via the easiest route – water pipes, the return wire, earth stake or a person.
Harmonic	multiples of the original frequency.
Homeostasis	equilibrium, balance/regulation.
Hormone	chemicals which circulate in the bloodstream and spread around the body to carry messages or signals to different parts of the body.
IARC	International Agency for Research on Cancer
ICNIRP	International Commission for Non-Ionizing Radiation Protection – EUROPE

| *In utero* | in the uterus, before birth. |

In utero — in the uterus, before birth.

In vitro — in glass.

In vivo — in a living body.

[*In vitro* (in glass) studies provide insights into the mechanisms underlying biological effects, whereas *in vivo* (in a living body) studies of animals and humans are considered to provide more convincing evidence of biological effects that have implications for adverse health consequences for people].

Ionising radiation — electromagnetic radiation with photon energy high enough to break molecular bonds and damage genetic material. Gamma rays and x-rays are examples.

Ionsphere — reflects certain electromagnetic frequencies much like a mirror reflects light and enables short-wave radio communication across the globe.

Leukemogen — a factor that is known or attributed to be a cause of leukaemia.

Lou Gehrig's disease — also called Amyotrophic lateral sclerosis (ALS), motor neuron disease. Is a progressive, fatal, neurodegenerative disease caused by the degeneration of motor neurons, the nerve cells in the central nervous system that control voluntary muscle movement. Messages to muscles cease.

Luteal phase — after ovulation and before the onset of menstruation.

LH — luteinizing hormone.

Mammary — pertaining to the breast.

MCF-7 cells — human oestrogen-responsive breast cancer cells.

Mechanism — step by step sequence – along a chain of causes.

mG — milliGauss (old measurement of a magnetic field). A milliGauss is a measure of ELF intensity, and is used to describe electromagnetic fields from appliances, power lines, interior electrical wiring etc.

Melatonin — a natural neurohormone produced by the pineal gland from serotonin that regulates the activity of the brain. Been shown to enhance the immune system, capable of neutralising the negative effects that stress, drugs and infections have on the immune system. Its roles are many including being a chronobiotic agent.

Meta-analysis — pooled results of individual, comparable studies.

MFs — magnetic fields.

MW — microwave. Technology that operates at this frequency includes: cell phones, microwaves, radar, telecommunications links, satellite communications, weather-observation equipment and medical diathermy. Because microwaves are also used for communication, RF and MW emissions overlap considerably. Microwave energy is within the radio frequency band of the electromagnetic spectrum and ranges from 300 MHz to 300 GHz.

Neurohormone — important hormone in the body.

NIEHS	The National Institute of Environmental Health Sciences (NIEHS/NIH) is one of the National Institutes of Health within the U.S. Department of Health and Human Services National Toxicology Program (NTP).
Nocturnal	occurring at night.
Non-ionising radiation	part of the electromagnetic spectrum extending from zero frequency to the frequencies of visible light.
NIER	Non-ionising electromagnetic radiation. Includes all radiations and fields of the electromagnetic spectrum that do not normally have sufficient energy to produce ionisation in matter.
Oncostatic	cancer suppressing.
Oscillating	having periodic vibrations.
Per se	on its own – not connected to another matter.
Pituitary Gland	the main endocrine gland often called "the master gland". Small hormone-producing gland in the brain which secretes substances necessary for basic life processes.
Plausible	apparently reasonable and valid, truthful.
Precautionary Principle	the 'Precautionary Principle' states when there are indications of possible adverse effects, though they remain uncertain, the risks from doing nothing may be far greater than the risks of taking action to control these exposures. The 'Precautionary Principle' shifts the burden of proof from those suspecting a risk to those who discount it.
Precursor	a process that precedes a later stage.
Pro bono	legal services free of charge for the public 'good'.
Prolactin	hormone produced by the pituitary gland in the brain that stimulates breast development and milk development.
Prospective	a study or clinical trial in which participants are identified and then followed forward in time.
Radiation	energy transmitted by waves that travels and spreads out as it goes.
Resonance	the tuning of a biological response to an external signal. Resonance can also be applicable to organs, tissues, or other body parts.
RFR	radiofrequency radiation. Higher frequency radiation used by communications systems. Used in technologies such as mobile communications, radios, TVs, paging antennae, computer. Measured in microwatts per square centimetre (μW/cm2).
Schumann Resonances	set of spectrum peaks in the extremely low frequency (ELF) portion of the Earth's electromagnetic field spectrum.
Sex hormone related cancers	breast, prostate, uterus, ovaries.
Spot measurements	average magnetic field over a period of seconds or minutes.
Stem cells	cells that can differentiate into many different cell types when subjected to the right biochemical signals. Cells from which all blood cells derive. Bone marrow is rich in stem cells.

Subharmonics	fractions of the original frequency.
Suprachiasmatic nucleus	SCN. Is a region of the brain, located in the hypothalamus that is responsible for controlling endogenous circadian rhythms.
SW	short wave.
T:	Tesla – alternative measurement of magnetic field: mT – millitesla µT – microtesla (Multiply microTesla by 10 to convert to milliGauss). 1 µT = 10mG 1.2µ T = 12mG 100 µT = 1 G
Tamoxifen	a drug used to treat breast cancer, and to prevent it in women who are at a high risk of developing breast cancer. Tamoxifen blocks the effects of the hormone oestrogen in the breast. In breast tumours that depend on oestrogen for growth, tamoxifen can prevent breast cancer cells from dividing and multiplying further by blocking the action of oestrogen. Currently the world's largest selling breast cancer treatment.
Time-weighted average	TWA. Over the course of a 24-hour period.
Transformer	converts electricity to a different voltage.
Transients	large, very brief increases in voltage. Distortions in the sine wave that occur when electrical equipment is switched on or off. They have the effect of creating a high frequency signal that is superimposed on the 50/60 Hz signal.
VDT	video display terminal.
VDU	video display units for computers, videos, TV and some measurement devices using cathode ray tubes.
(µW/cm2)	radiofrequency radiation in terms of power density is measured in microwatts per centimetre squared and abbreviated (µW/cm2). Measurement used for emissions from wireless facilities, and when describing ambient RF in the environment.
WI-FI	stands for wireless fidelity. WI-FI systems create zones of wireless RF that allow access to wireless internet for computers, internet phone access and other wireless services. The range of typical WI-FI systems is about 300 feet.
WI-MAX	stands for "Wireless Interoperability for Microwave Access" and is a telecommunications technology aimed at providing wireless data over long distances. Like WI-FI, WIMAX systems are designed to provide wireless access but over much broader geographic areas, with some systems transmitting signal up to 10 miles. Higher levels of RF are produced at the wireless transmission facilities than for WI-FI.
X-ray	penetrating, ionising electromagnetic radiation.

Appendix A

THE ELECTROMAGNETIC SPECTRUM

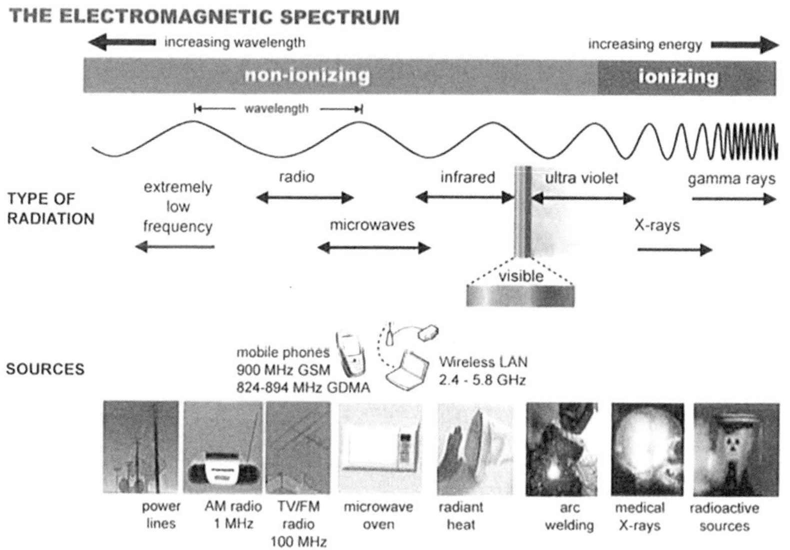

Taken from www.adm.monash.edu.au/ohse/safety-topics/em-spectrum.html

Appendix B

ELF EMF and RF EMF

As more people are seeking to gain further understanding of electromagnetic radiation an explanation of the difference between the fields from powerlines and the fields from mobile phone towers – radiofrequency fields (RF EMF) – is as follows:

EMR
Electromagnetic Radiation

ELF EMF	RF EMF
Powerlines	Mobile phones
Sub-stations	Mobile phone masts
Electrical equipment	TV, radio and other
Electrical appliances	broadcast antennas
Wiring in buildings	Wireless internet

At ELF frequencies the term EMFs means "electric and magnetic fields", meaning that the separate fields exist. At radio-frequencies (RF) the term EMFs means "electromagnetic fields".

For more sources of EMR refer to Appendix D.

MOBILE PHONES

The Russian National Commission on Non-Ionizing Radiation Protection (RNCNIRP) not only advises against mobile phone use by children but they specifically state that people with neurological conditions should not use mobile phones as it could worsen the symptoms.

For more in-depth information on mobile phone technologies refer to The Benevento Resolution in Chapter 7 and The BioInitiative Report in Chapter 8.

TELECOMMUNICATIONS MASTS

For the communities who are uneasy and resisting the installation of telecommunications masts nearby, the following information is included:

In a 1994/1995 court-case against a telecommunications company in the Planning Tribunal in New Zealand, Dr Cherry appeared for the local residents who won the case. The court decision set the public exposure level at $2\mu W/cm^2$ based on evidence of childhood leukaemia at $2.4\mu W/cm^2$, rejecting the request by the telecommunications company for a $200\mu W/cm^2$ public exposure standard. Dr Cherry also found evidence of effects well below $2\mu W/cm^2$ pointing to zero exposure as the level of no effect.

Dr Cherry recommended an outdoor public exposure limit at the boundary of properties of $0.1\mu W/cm^2$ the city of Salzburg cell site limit.

When telecommunications equipment was constructed at the Brunswick Community Services building in Victoria, Australia, workers stipulated that the telecommunications company adhere to levels set by Dr Cherry.

The BioInitiative Report August 2007 recommends "a precautionary limit" of $0.1\mu W/cm^2$ (0.6V/m) for RF exposures where "people live, work and go to school." *(Summary for the Public)*

Also refer:

- the Salzburg Resolution on Mobile Telecommunication Base Stations, Salzburg, June 2000.
- the Freiburger Appeal, Germany, October 2002.

BROADCAST ANTENNAS

In the largest and most detailed study of AM radio radiation to date, a team led by Mina Ha of South Korea's Dankook University in South Korea found that children living within 2km of an AM transmitter had more than twice the risk of developing leukaemia, compared to those living more than 20km away. Ha's study included 31 AM stations.

(Refer Mina Ha, Hyoungjune Im, Mihye Lee, Hyun Joo Kim, Byung-Chan Kim, Yoon-Myoung Gimm and Jeong-Ki Pack *Radio-Frequency Radiation Exposure from AM Radio Transmitters and Childhood Leukemia and Brain Cancer*, American Journal of Epidemiology 2007 166(3):270-279). (Reported in *Microwave News* July 13 2007).

WIRELESS INTERNET – WI-FI, WIMAX

Refer to:

- The Benevento Resolution September 2006
- The BioInitiative Report August 2007

Following on from the release of the scientific review The BioInitiative Report in September 2007, Europe's top environmental watchdog – the EU's European Environment Agency (EEA) is calling for immediate action to reduce exposure to radiation from WI-FI (and mobile phones and their masts).

For more information on the current scientific opinion in relation to EMR of some of the world's leading scientists refer to the recently signed Benevento Resolution (September 2006) and The BioInitiative Report (August 2007).

Various websites throughout the world continually update information on EMR. These include:

www.electric-fields.bris.ac.uk

www.microwavenews.com

www.powerwatch.org.uk

www.energyfields.org

www.emfacts.com

At www.energyfields.org find the B Blake Levitt and Theresa Morrow article *Electrosmog: What Price Convenience*.

Appendix C

Electrohypersensitivity

From presentations at "Understanding Electrohypersensitivity Symposium", Netherlands – December 8, 2006

Top ten complaints:

1. fatigue
2. concentration/memory problems
3. insomnia
4. tinnitus
5. pressure in/out head
6. headache
7. vertigo
8. blurred vision
9. skin rashes
10. pain

Top ten hazards:

1. DECT phones
2. waterbeds
3. alarm clocks
4. wireless networks
5. children's mobile phones
6. magnetrons (in microwave ovens)
7. electrical installations
8. electric blankets
9. electronic stove
10. TV

Main sources in the office:
1. transformer
2. hardware
3. wireless networks
4. wireless connections
5. Bluetooth headsets
6. lighting and cabling
7. mobile phones
8. electronic cars

Main sources outside:
1. base stations
2. phones in bus/trains
3. high tension wires
4. trains and stations
5. radio and TV
6. radar
7. promotional signs

For more information contact **www.ukselfhelp.info/circuit**

Sourced from: *EMR AND HEALTH* (Vol.3 No 1.2007 p.9)

Appendix D

Sources of Electromagnetic Radiation (EMR) include:

"Laptop computers used from the mains; televisions; battery operated appliances; fish tank heaters or lights; telephones; answer phones and faxes, mobile and digital cordless phones; refrigerators; freezers; electric cookers (including induction hobs); vacuum cleaners etc; photocopiers; signalling circuits for cable TV; lamps with attached or built-in transformers; dimmer switches; fire/burglar alarms; fluorescent lights; low energy, mercury and sodium light; fuse panels; pylons, power lines, substations; underground electric cables; water and gas pipelines with associated net currents; uninterrupted power supply (UPS); electric fields due to house wiring; hearing-aid induction loops; electrical noise in trains; underground trains, trams, buses and cars; mobile phone base station masts; fan rooms; high-frequency amplitude-modulated light; heat; VDUs; electronic medical procedures, especially MRI scan; daylight, weather changes; laser beams in supermarkets; electronic 'anti-theft' tagging scanners at the exits to many department stores; thyristors; some new up-market cars, especially those with RF communications systems."

Sourced from *EMR AND HEALTH* – (Vol 1 No 4, 2005, p. 2)

Appendix E

Breast Cancer and Radiation

Previously it was thought that the gonadal (female – ovaries, male – testes) organs were the most sensitive part of the body to radiation. Breast tissue is now regarded as even more sensitive to radiation.

The electromagnetic spectrum, as we know it, is comprised of ionising radiation and non-ionising radiation.

It has been known for many decades that ionising radiation can cause breast cancer, both by directly damaging DNA and by disrupting normal cellular and intra-cellular processes. There is no safe dose and the genetic damage accumulates over a lifetime. Ionising radiation includes:

- Gamma rays – nuclear bombs, nuclear power plants.

  Gamma radiation is a known genotoxic agent. Survivors from the Hiroshima and Nagasaki atomic bomb were studied and in 1968, C.K. Wanebo and colleagues – following on from previous work by Ian MacKenzie (1965) – published confirmatory evidence of human breast-cancer induction by ionising radiation. The induction of breast-cancer by ionising radiation was later confirmed and quantified.

  At the Second World Breast Cancer Conference, Ottawa, 1999, it was reported that people who live near nuclear power plants are more likely to develop breast cancer and other types of cancer. Dr Jay Gould, director of the Radiation and Public Health Project in the US stated his own research in Long Island, New York, shows that there are "extraordinarily high" levels of female cancers including breast cancer within 16 kilometers of a reactor. Long Island also has an unusually high rate of rare childhood bone cancer.

- Medical X-rays, CT Scans, Mammograms

  Dr John W Gofman, PhD, in *Preventing Breast Cancer: The Story of a Major, Proven, Preventable Cause of This Disease*, shows that past exposure to ionising radiation – primarily medical x-rays – is responsible for about 75 percent of the breast cancer problem in the United States. A CT scan exposes patients to more radiation than a standard X-ray – CT scans provide more diagnostic information but the dose is higher. Multi-slice CT scanners deliver higher doses of radiation than single-slice scanners.

Even though mammography is seen as the 'gold' standard in testing for breast cancer because of its accuracy, mammography also exposes women to ionising radiation. The necessity of having an annual mammogram for pre-menopausal women is now being seriously questioned. The pre-menopausal breast is highly sensitive to radiation, a fact that has been known for over three decades.

The challenge of mammography is producing higher quality mammography images while trying to keep patient radiation dose low as radiation can cause breast cancer as well as detect it.

The breast consists of three different tissues: fibrous tissue, glandular tissue, and adipose tissue. The tissue most sensitive to radiation is glandular tissue and pre-menopausal women have breasts composed mainly of fibrous and glandular tissue surrounded by a thin layer of fat which means these breasts are dense and difficult to image. More imaging represents more radiation. In post-menopausal women, the glandular tissue turns to fat. The newer diagnostic tools for first-line screening for breast health include the CRT-2000 and Digital Thermal Imaging (DITI).

The indiscriminate use of ionising radiation has had devastating consequences on individuals and society as a whole. For more information on this controversial issue refer to the views expressed by Dr Samuel S. Epstein, Chairman of the Cancer Prevention Coalition and Professor Emeritus of Environmental and Occupational Medication, University of Illinois School of Public Health, Chicago and The XaHP – The X-rays and Health Project – website.

Radiation exposure in the ionising part of the electromagnetic spectrum is the only established external exposure that can cause leukaemia. The non-ionising part of the electromagnetic spectrum is now also implicated.

Radiation exposure in the ionising part of the electromagnetic spectrum is the only established external exposure that can cause breast cancer. Is it such a surprise when the same disease risk is demonstrated to be in the non-ionising spectrum of which extremely low frequency electromagnetic fields (ELF EMF) are a part?

Low dose exposures over time as well as acute high dosages are of concern in regard to ionising radiation. This concern has extended to ELF EMF. It is critical that the public be informed and strategies be implemented that limit ELF EMF exposure in the quest to prevent breast cancer.

Appendix F

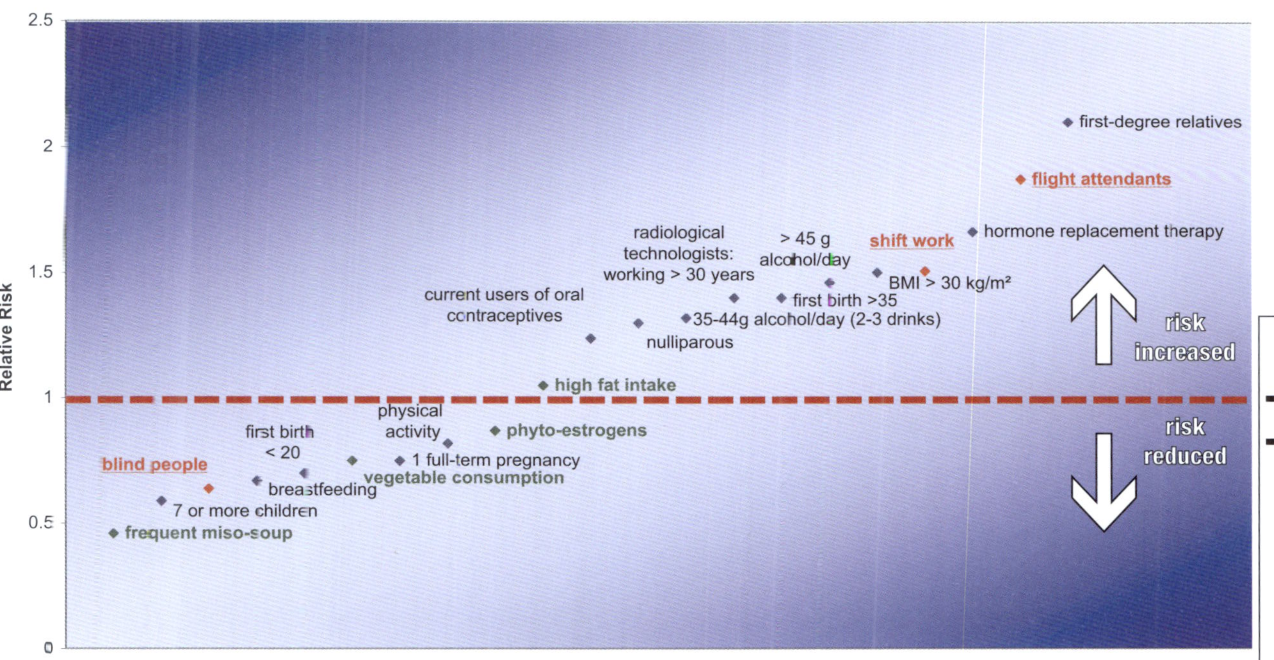

Possible chronobiological factors are marked in RED, nutritional factors in GREEN, others in BLUE.

Appendix G

Further Investigation

According to Dr Richard Stevens, EMF and/or light-at-night and its effects on melatonin may affect the risk for breast cancer in three ways:

- if melatonin suppresses reproductive hormones, such as oestrogen, melatonin suppression could allow oestrogen levels to rise, stimulating growth in breast tissue and oestrogen-responsive breast cancers.

- if melatonin suppresses breast cancer cell growth directly, reduction in melatonin could allow breast cancers to grow more rapidly.

- if melatonin boosts immune function, a change in melatonin could compromise the immune system's ability to control cell transformation.

The following graph originally proposed by Dr Richard Stevens and updated to include the pituitary link is presented by Dr Thomas Erren in *The Melatonin Hypothesis: Breast Cancer and Use of Electric Power*.

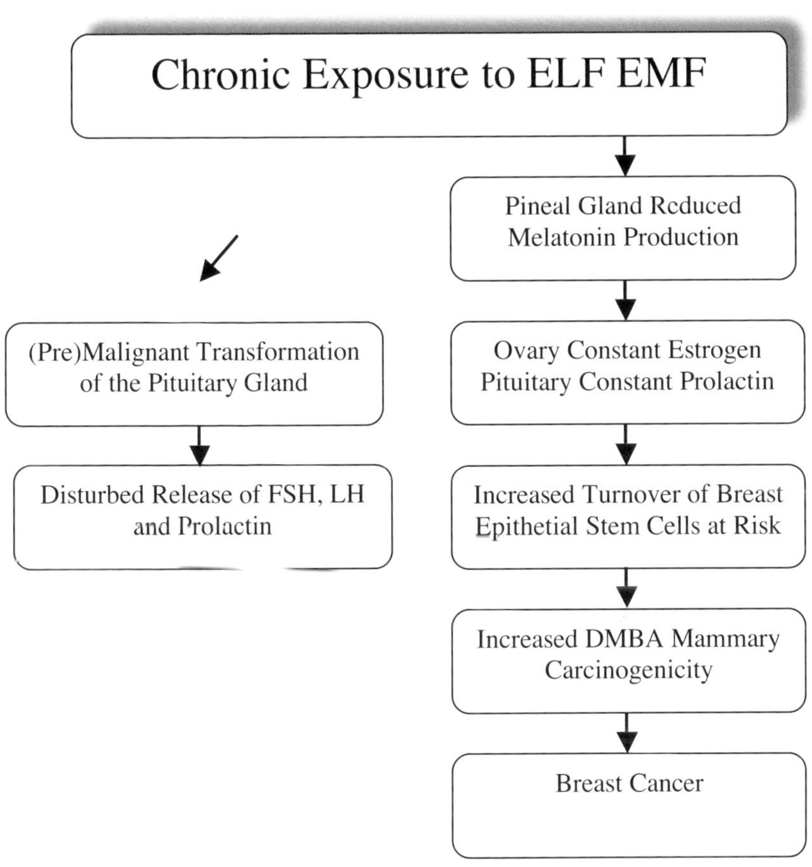

"Hypothetical hormone-mediated mammary carcinogenesis. Model adapted from Stevens (1987) and modified by findings of Floderus *et al.* (1994). Proposed "functional pinealectomy" by chronic exposure to ELF EMF as an etiologic factor for breast cancer in rats. Hypothetically, long term exposure to ELF EMF causes a (pre)malignant transformation of the pituitary gland, which may result in cancer of hormonal target organs like the breast and/or cancer of the gland itself".[i]

[i] Erren in Stevens, Wilson, Anderson 1997, p.705

Appendix H

ELF EMF / RF EMF / MW for Healing Purposes

Research has been ongoing for centuries on using ELF fields and radiation for healing purposes. The body's healing process is controlled by minute electrical signals – even cancer cells conduct electricity. Samuel Hahnemann (1755-1843), the founder of homeopathy, reasoned that what can create disease can also heal depending on dose and application.

The latest research in this field that may prove to be an effective cancer therapy that does not kill dormant cells is the work of small high-tech Israeli company NovoCure. NovoCure has used weak electric fields to stunt the growth of cancer cells either by slowing down their growth or killing them off. *Microwave News* reported the observed effect is frequency dependent and clearly non-thermal, according to the NovoCure team.

(Proceedings of the National Academy of Sciences (PNAS) June 12 2007).

Used with intention and correctly within specific parameters, ELF EMF can be effective treatments for bone repair and wound healing. Dr Robert O. Becker was nominated for a Nobel Prize for his pioneering work on healing bone fractures and oedema with externally applied ELF electromagnetic fields. Twice nominated for a Nobel Prize in Medicine, Dr Becker was one of the first medical pioneers to study natural electrical currents in the human body and to caution about electro-pollution. The scientific literature in regard to pulsed EMF, which can stimulate bone cell growth, is extensive, showing that pulsed EMF have been tuned to resonate with biological processes. The FDA approved pulsed EMF for use in bone healing in 1979.

More recently Min Zhao and an international team of researchers found that by applying artificial fields to wounds they could speed up or inhibit the repair process, depending on the attributes of the field. (Zhao, M *et al.*, Nature 442, 457-460; 27 July 2006).

Dr Cherry contended that the therapeutic use of picoTesla ELF fields in the successful treatment of a range of neurological diseases, specifically Parkinson's disease and MS, confirms the magneto-sensitivity of the human pineal and the role of melatonin as the biological mechanism for this therapy.

Even though these therapies support the contention that these fields are bioactive there is still strong resistance to implicate ELF EMF in disease processes.

As far back as 1990 Dr Robert O. Becker stated: "There does seem to be a direct link between suicide, depression, and functions of the pineal gland".[i] It is the understanding of electromagnetic therapies as clinically accepted forms of therapy for such diverse diseases as uni-polar depression, Parkinson's disease, sleep disorders and the treatment of debilitating chronic and acute pain that will pave the way for noninvasive forms of treatment of many disease processes.

Another example is the use of radio-wave hyperthermia for prostate cancer. Used in Europe this treatment passes electromagnetic waves from a transmitter through the patient to a receiving plate.

An example of using radio waves as a therapy in the treatment of cancer is the work of Dr John Holt, in Perth, Western Australia. In working with high frequency radiation (used in conjunction with glycolytic blocking agents) this microwave therapy involves exposing cancer cells to 434 MHz ultra high frequency radio waves, a frequency also used in Europe for decades. Since Dr Holt's retirement, the privately funded Radiowave Therapy Research Institute in Claremont, Western Australia has taken over Dr Holt's treatment methods, treating patients and collating the research. For cancer treatment enquiries telephone (08) 9285 4000 in Australia, international +61 8 92854000.

The intriguing area of further research into controlled EMFs with intent for healing purposes – as a noninvasive technology that does not damage healthy cells in the process – is continuing.

i   Becker 1990, p.264

Appendix I

Signees of The Benevento Resolution

We, the undersigned scientists, agree to assist in the promotion of EMF research and the development of strategies to protect public health through the wise application of the precautionary principle.

Signed:

Fiorella Belpoggi, European Foundation for Oncology & Environmental Sciences, B. Ramazzini, Bologna, Italy

Carl F. Blackman, President, Bioelectromagnetics Society (1990-91), Raleigh, NC, USA

Martin Blank, Department of Physiology, Columbia University, New York, USA

Natalia Bobkova, Institute of Cell Biophysics, Pushchino, Moscow Region

Francesco Boella, National Institute Prevention & Worker Safety, Venice, Italy

Zhaojin Cao, National Institute Environmental Health, Chinese Center for Disease Control, China

Sandro D. Allessandro, Physician, Mayor of Benevento, Italy, (2001-2006)

Enrico D. Emilia, National Institute for Prevention and Worker Safety, Monteporzio, Italy

Emilio Del Giuduice, National Institute for Nuclear Physics, Milan, Italy

Antonella De Ninno, Italian National Agency for Energy, Environment & Technology, Frascati, Italy

Alvaro A. De Sallas, Universidade Federal do Rio Grande do Sul, Porto Alegre, Brazil

Livio Giuliani, East Veneto & South Triol, National Institute Prevention & Worker Safety, Camerino Universit

Yury Grigoryev, Institute of Biophysics; Chairman, Russian National Committee NIERP

Settimo Grimaldi, Institute Neurobiology & Molecular Medicine, National Research, Rome, Italy

Lennart Hardell, Department of Oncology, University Hospital, Orebro, Sweden

Magda Havas, Environmental & Resource Studies, Trent University, Ontario, Canada

Gerard Hyland, Warwick University, UK; International Institute Biophysics, Germany; EM Radiation Trust, UK

Olle Johansson, Experimental Dermatology Unit, Neuroscience Department, Karolinska Institute, Sweden

Michael Kundi, Head, Institute Environmental Health, Medical University of Vienna, Austria

Henry C. Lai, Department of Bioengineering, University of Washington, Seattle, USA

Mario Ledda, Institute Neurobiology & Molecular Medicine, National Council for Research, Rome, Italy

Yi-Ping Lin, Center of Health Risk Assessment & Policy, National Taiwan University, Taiwan

Antonella Lisi, Institute Neurobiology & Molecular Medicine, National Research Council, Rome, Italy

Fiorenzo Marinelli, Institute of Immunocytology, National Research Council, Bologna, Italy

Elihu Richter, Head, Occupational & Environmental Medicine, Hebrew University-Hadassah, Israel

Emanuela Rosola, Institute Neurobiology & Molecular Medicine, National Research Council, Rome, Italy

Leif Salford, Chairman, Department of Neurosurgery, Lund University, Sweden

Nesrin Seyhan, Head, Department of Biophysics; Director, Gazi NIRP Center, Ankara, Turkey

Morando Soffritti, Scientific Director, European Foundation for Oncology & Environmental Sciences, B Ramazzini, Bologna, Italy

Stanislaw Szmigielski, Military Institute of Hygiene and Epidemiology, Warsaw, Poland

Mikhail Zhadin, Institute of Cell Biophysics, Pushchino, Moscow Region

Additional signers after September 19, 2006:

Igor Y. Belyaev, Department of Genetics, Microbiology and Toxicology, Arrhenius Laboratories for Natural Sciences, Stockholm University, Stockholm, Sweden

William J. Bruno, PhD., Theoretical Biophysics, awarded by Department of Physics, University of California at Berkeley, USA

Mauro Cristaldi, Dip, B.A.U. Universita degli Studi "La Sapienza", Roma, Italia

Suleyman Dasdag, Biophysics Department of Medical School, Dicle University, Diyarbakir, Turkey

Sandy Doull, Consultant, Noel Arnold & Associates, Box Hill, Victoria, Australia

Christos D. Georgio, Assoc. Professor of Biochemistry, Department of Biology, University of Patras, Greece

Reba Goodman, Prof. Emeritus, Clinical Pathology, Columbia University, New York, New York, USA

Luisa Anna Ieradi, Istituto per lo Studio degli Ecosistemi C.N.R., Roma, Italia

Angelo Gino Lewis, Professor Emeritus, Environmental Oncology, Padua University, Italy

Lukas H. Margaritis, Professor of Cell Biology and Radiobiology, Athens University, Athens, Greece

Vera Markovic, Faculty of Electrical Engineering, University of Nis, Serbia

Gerd Oberfeld, Federal Salzburg Government, National Medical Management, Public Health Hygiene and Environmental Health, Salzburg, Austria

Jerry L. Phillips, Professor, University of Colorado, Colorado Springs, USA

Zamir Shalita, Consultant on Electromagnetic Hazards, Ramat Gan, Israel

E. Stanton Maxey, M.D. retired surgeon, Fayetteville, Arkansas

Ion Udroiu, Dip. B.A.U., Università degli Studi "La Sapienza", Roma, Italia

Mehmet Zeyrek, Professor, Physics Department, Middle East Technical University, Ankara, Turkey

Stelios A Zinelis, M.D., Vice President, Hellenic Cancer Society, Cefallonia, Greece

Additional signers who are qualified but have not published EMF papers or published prior to 2000.

Andrew Goldsworthy, Lecturer in biology (retired), Imperial College London, United Kingdom

Sarah J. Starkey, PhD, Neuroscience, University of London, London, United Kingdom

Appendix J

The List of Bioinitiative Participants:

Organizing Committee Members –

Carl F. Blackman*, PhD Founder, Former President and Full Member of the Bioelectromagnetics Society Raleigh, NC USA *opinions expressed are not necessarily those of his employer, the US Environmental Protection Agency

Martin Blank, PhD Associate Professor Former President and Full Member of Bioelectromagnetics Society, Dept of Physiology College of Physicians and Surgeons Columbia University, New York, NY USA

Professor Michael Kundi, PhD Full Member of the Bioelectromagnetics Society Institute of Environmental Health, Medical University of Vienna, Vienna, Austria

Cindy Sage, MA Owner Full Member Bioelectromagnetics Society, Sage Associates Santa Barbara, CA USA

Participants –

David O. Carpenter, MD Director, Institute for Health and the Environment University at Albany East Campus Rensselaer, NY USA

Zoreh Davanipour, DVM PhD Friends Research Institute Los Angeles, CA USA

David Gee, Program Chair Coordinator Emerging Issues and Scientific Liaison Strategic Knowledge and Innovation European Environmental Agency Copenhagen, Denmark

Lennart Hardell, MD PhD Professor Department of Oncology University Hospital Orebro, Sweden

Olle Johansson, PhD Associate Professor The Experimental Dermatology Unit Department of Neuroscience Karolinska Institute Stockholm, Sweden

Henry Lai, PhD Department of Bioengineering University of Washington Seattle, Washington USA

Bibliography

Armstrong   B, Professor, 2006 *Breast Cancer at the ABC Toowong Queensland: Third Progress Report,* Independent Review and Scientific Investigation Panel, AUS

Becker,   Robert O, Dr, 1990 *Cross Currents*, Tarcher Putnam, US

Blackman,   C F, Benane, S G, House, D E, 2001 *The Influence of 1.2 microT, 60 Hz Magnetic Fields on Melatonin and Tamoxifen-induced Inhibition of MCF-7 cell growth.* Bioelectromagnetics, 22: 122–128

Blask,   D E, Brainard G C, Dauchy R T, Hanifin J P, Davidson L K, Krause J A, Sauer L A, Rivera-Bermudez M A, Dubocovich M L, Jasser S A, Lynch D T, Rollag M D, Zalatan F, *Melatonin-Depleted Blood from Premenopausal Women Exposed to Light at Night Stimulates Growth of Human Breast Cancer Xenografts in Nude Rats* American Association for Cancer Research, USA

Brodeur,   P, 1995 *The Great Power-line Cover-Up: How the Utilities and the Government are Trying to Hide the Cancer Hazards Posed by Electromagnetic Fields*, Little Brown & Company (Canada) Ltd, USA

Borysenko,   J, Dr PhD, 1996 *A Woman's Life: The Biology, Psychology and Spirituality of the Feminine Life Cycle* Berkley Publishing Group, USA

Bushong,   S C, 2004 Radiologic *Science for Technologists*, Elsevier Mosby, USA

Carpenter,   D Dr, Sage C MA (eds), 2007 *The BioInitiative Report: A Rationale for a Biologically-based Public Exposure Standard for Electromagnetic Fields* (ELF and RF) The BioInitiative Working Group, USA

Carpenter,   D Dr, Sage C MA (eds), 2007 *Section 17 – Key Scientific Evidence and Public Health Policy Recommendations The BioInitiative Report: A Rationale for a Biologically-based Public Exposure Standard for Electromagnetic Fields* (ELF and RF) The BioInitiative Working Group, USA

Cherry,   N, Dr O.N.Z.M., 1999 *Criticism of the Proposal to Adopt the ICNIRP Guidelines for Cellsites in New Zealand: ICNIRP Guideline Critique*, Lincoln University, New Zealand

Cherry,   N, Dr O.Z.N.M., 1999 *Electromagnetic Radiation Causes Cancer: The Implications for Breast Cancer*, World Conference on Breast Cancer, Ottawa, Canada, 26-31 July

Cherry,   N, Dr O.Z.N.M., 2000 April 25 *Cherry on Safe Exposure Levels*, Lincoln University, New Zealand

Cherry,   N, Dr O.Z.N.M., 2000 June *Evidence that Electromagnetic Radiation is Genotoxic: The Implications for the Epidemiology of Cancer and Cardiac, Neurological and Reproductive Effects*, For presentations in May to NZ Parliament and June 2000 in

Italy, Australia, Ireland and at the European Parliament in Brussels, New Zealand

Cherry,   N, Dr O.Z.N.M., 2000 September 8 *Health Effects of Electromagnetic Radiation: Evidence for the Australian Senate Committee* New Zealand

Cherry,   N, Dr O.Z.N.M., 2001 May 1 *Evidence that Electromagnetic Fields from High Voltage Powerlines and in Buildings, are Hazardous to Human Health, Especially to Young Children*, Environmental Management and Design Division, Lincoln University, New Zealand

Davanipour,   Z, DVM, PhD, Sobel E PhD, 2007 *EMF & Melatonin: Alzheimers Disease & Breast Cancer. Section 12 – Evidence for Effects on Melatonin: Alzheimer's Disease and Breast Cancer*, The BioInitiative Working Group, USA

Doull,   A, 2001 *Expert Witness Report*, Planning & Environment Court 2064 of 2001, Brisbane, AUS

Ellwood,   M Professor, 2001 *Statement of Evidence*, Planning & Environment Court 2601 of 2001, Brisbane, AUS

Epstein,   S MD, Bertell, R, PhD., GNSH, Seaman, B, 2001 *Danger and Unreliability of Mammography: Breast Examination is a Safe, Effective and Practical Alternative*, International Journal of Health Services, Vol 31, Number 3, Pages 605-615, Baywood Publishing Co., Inc. USA

Erren,   T C Dr, 1997 *Epidemiologic Studies of EMF and Breast Cancer Risk: A Biologically Based Overview* in Richard G Stevens, Bary W Wilson and Larry E Anderson (eds) *The Melatonin Hypothesis: Breast Cancer and Use of Electric Power*, Columbus: Battelle Press, USA

Erren,   T C Dr, 2005 *Letters to the Editor* Am J Epidemiol 2005;162:389–395

Fedrowitz,   M, Kamino K, Loscher W, 2004 *Significant Differences in the Effects of Magnetic Field Exposure on 7,12-Dimethylbenz(a)anthracene-Induced Mammary Carcinogenesis in Two Substrains of Sprague-Dawley Rats*, Cancer Research Jan 1;64: 243–251

Feytching,   M, Forss'en U, 2006 *Electromagnetic Fields and Female Breast Cancer* Cancer Causes Control 17:553–558 DOI 10.1007/s10552-005-9008-3

Forss'en,   UM, Rutqvist LE, Ahlbom A, *et al.*, 2005 *Occupational Magnetic Fields and Female Breast Cancer: a Case-Control Study Using Swedish Population Registers and New Exposure Data*. Am J Epidemiol 2005;161:250–9.

Gofman,   J Dr PhD, 1996 *Preventing Breast Cancer: The Story of a Major, Proven, Preventable Cause of This Disease*, C.N.R. Book Division, Committee for Nuclear Responsibility Inc. USA

Graham,   C and Gibertini, M, 1997 *Human Exposure to Magnetic Fields: Effects on Melatonin, Hormones, and Immunity* in Richard G Stevens, Bary W Wilson and Larry E Anderson (eds) *The Melatonin Hypothesis: Breast Cancer and Use of Electric Power*, Columbus: Battelle Press, USA

Gray,   J PhD (Ed) 2008 *State of the Evidence 2008: The Connection Between Breast Cancer and the Environment*, Breast Cancer Fund USA

Ha   *et al.*, 2007 *Radio-Frequency Radiation Exposure from AM Radio Transmitters and Childhood Leukemia and Brain Cancer* Am J of Epidemiology Advance Access USA

Hansen,   N H, 1997 *Understanding Dose: Implications for Bioelectromagnetics Research* in Richard G Stevens, Bary W Wilson and Larry E Anderson (eds) *The Melatonin Hypothesis: Breast Cancer and Use of Electric Power*, Columbus: Battelle Press, USA

Havas,   M BSc PhD, 2008 *Dirty Electricity Elevates Blood Sugar Among Electrically Sensitive Diabetics and May Explain Brittle Diabetes,* Electromagnetic Biology and Medicine, 27:135-146.

Havas,   M BSc PhD, 2007 *Analysis of Health and Environmental Effects of Proposed San Francisco Earthlink Wi-Fi Network*, Trent University, Canada

Havas,   M BSc PhD, 2006 *Electromagnetic Hypersensitivity: Biological Effects of Dirty Electricity with Emphasis on Diabetes and Multiple Sclerosis*, Electromagnetic Biology and Medicine, 25:259-268 Canada.

Havas,   M BSc PhD, 2001 *Health Effects Associated with Power Lines* presented to Steering Committee, Public Hearing on the SW Metro Transmission Line USA, Trent University, Canada

Havas,   M BSc PhD, 2000 *Biological Effects of Non-Ionizing Electromagnetic Energy: A Critical Review of the Reports by the US National Research Council of the US National Institute of Environmental Health Sciences as They Relate to the Broad Realm of EMF Bioeffects*, Environ 8:173-253, NRC Research Press, Canada

Havas,   M BSc PhD, Stetzer D, 2004 *Dirty Electricity and Electrical Hypersensitivity: Five Case Studies*, World Health Organization Workshop in Electrical Hypersensitivity 25-26 October, Prague, Czech Republic

Henshaw,   D L Professor, 2007 *Powerline Report Fails to Protect the Public Against Health Risks* Human Radiation Effects Group UK

Henshaw,   D L Professor, 2005 *Comment on the Draper Report* Human Radiation Effects Group UK

Henshaw,   D L Professor, O'Carroll, M.J., 2007 *Response from Professor Denis L Henshaw and Professor Mike J O'Carroll – Australian Government Australian Radiation Protection and Nuclear Safety Agency Draft Radiation Protection Standard for Exposure Limits to Electric and Magnetic Fields 0Hz – 2 kHz*, www.electric-fields.bris.ac UK

Henshaw,   D L Professor, Reiter R J Dr, 2004 *Do Magnetic Fields Cause Increased Risk of Childhood Leukemia via Melatonin Disruption?* The World Health Organisation International EMF Project Workshop on Sensitivity to Children to EMF, Istanbul, Turkey.

Hollingsworth, E, 2004 *Take Control of Your Health and Escape the Sickness Industry*, Eighth Edition, Empowerment Press International AUS

Juutilainen *et al*, 2006 *Do Extremely Low frequency Magnetic Fields Enhance the Effects of Environmental Carcinogens? A meta-analysis of experimental studies* Int J. Radiat. Biol., Vol. 82, No. 1, January p. 1-12.

Kabuto   *et al.*, 2006 *Childhood Leukemia and Magnetic Fields in Japan: A Case-Control Study of Childhood Leukemia and Residential Power-Frequency Magnetic Fields in Japan*, International Journal of Cancer Vol. 119, Issue 3, p. 643-650

Kundi,   M Professor, 2007 *Section 11 – Evidence for Childhood Cancers (Leukemia) The BioInitiative Report: A Rationale for a Biologically – based Public Exposure Standard for Electromagnetic Fields (ELF and RF)*, The Bioinitiative Working Group, USA

Lamb,   R 2002 *Summary Report – Energex Limited V Logan City Council V Others Planning & Environment Court Appeal* 2604 of 2001, BEES AUS

Lai,   H Dr, 2007 *Section 6 – Evidence for Genotoxic Effects (RFR AND ELF Genotoxicity) The BioInitiative Report: A Rationale for a Biologically – based Public Exposure Standard for Electromagnetic Fields (ELF and RF)*, The Bioinitiative Working Group, USA

Lee,   J M Jnr, Stormshak, F, Thompson, J, Hess, D L, Hefeneider, S,1997 *Studies of Melatonin, Cortisol, Progesterone, and Interleukin-1 in Sheep Exposed to EMF from a 500-kV Transmission Line* in Richard G Stevens, Bary W Wilson and Larry E Anderson (eds) *The Melatonin Hypothesis: Breast Cancer and Use of Electric Power*, Columbus: Battelle Press, USA

Levitt,   B Blake, 1995 *Electromagnetic Fields: A consumer's guide to the issues and how to protect ourselves*, A Harvest Original, USA

Liburdy,   R P, and Harland, J D, 1997 *Magnetic fields, Melatonin, Tamoxifen, and Human Breast Cancer Cell Growth* in Richard G Stevens, Bary W Wilson and Larry E Anderson (eds) *The Melatonin Hypothesis: Breast Cancer and Use of Electric Power*, Columbus: Battelle Press, USA

Liburdy,   R P, and Loscher, W, 1997 *Laboratory Studies on Extremely Low Frequency (50/60-Hz) Magnetic Fields and Carcinogenesis* in Richard G Stevens, Bary W Wilson and Larry E Anderson (eds) *The Melatonin Hypothesis: Breast Cancer and Use of Electric Power*, Columbus: Battelle Press, USA

Liburdy,   R P, Sloma, T R, Sokolic, R, Yaswen, P, 1993 *ELF Magnetic Fields, Breast Cancer, and Melatonin: 60 Hz Fields Block Melatonin's Oncostatic Action on ER and Breast Cancer Cell Proliferation*. J. Pineal Research, 14: 89–97

Loscher,   W, 2000 *Laboratory Studies on Magnetic Fields, Melatonin and Cancer* Low frequency EMF, Visible Light, Melatonin and Cancer International Symposium, May 4-5 2000, University of Cologne, Germany

Loscher,   W, and Mevissen, M, 1997 *Magnetic Fields and Breast Cancer: Experimental Studies on the Melatonin Hypothesis* in Richard G Stevens, Bary W Wilson and Larry E Anderson (eds) *The Melatonin Hypothesis: Breast Cancer and Use of Electric Power*, Columbus: Battelle Press, USA.

McLean,   L, *EMR and Health,* EMR Australia Pty Ltd, AUS

              2008 Vol 4. No 2.   *Australia's New Standard: Details of Australia's first standard for electrical (ELF) exposure have been made available to the public for the first time, EMR and Health,* AUS

2007 Vol 3. No 1. *Electrohypersensitivity – a Modern Syndrome*
2006 Vol 2. No 4. *News from Around the Globe*
2006 Vol 2. No 2. *Powerlines and Childhood Leukemia*
2006 Vol 2. No 3. *Cancer – a Conductor*
2006 Vol 2. No 3. *Body's Healing Fields*
2005 Vol 1. No 4. *Electrosensitivity – New UK Report*
2005 Vol 1. No 4. *Radiowaves as Therapy*
2002 Vol 1. No 3. *Research News*

McLean, L, 2002 *What's the Buzz*, Scribe Publishers, AUS

Megdal S P, Kroenke C H, Laden F *et al*. Pukkala E, and Schernhammer E S, 2005 *Night Work and Breast Cancer Risk: A systematic review and meta-analysis*, Eur J Cancer 41:2023-2032.

Milham, S, 2004 *A Cluster of Male Breast Cancer in Office Workers*, AM J Med, Vol 46. No 1.

Milham, S MD MPH, Morgan LL BS, 2008 *A new electromagnetic exposure metric: high frequency voltage transients associated with increased cancer incidence in teachers in a California school*, AM J Ind Med, May 29; 51: (8) 579-586, PMID:18512243

Miller, D L, 1997 *Overview of Electromagnetic Field Exposure and Dosimetry* in Richard G Stevens, Bary W Wilson and Larry E Anderson (eds) *The Melatonin Hypothesis: Breast Cancer and Use of Electric Power*, Columbus: Battelle Press, USA

Morgan, L, 2006 *High Frequency Transients on Electrical Wiring: A Missing Link to Increasing Diabetes and Asthma?* Director, Central Brain Tumor Registry of the United States, American Academy of Environmental Medicine 39th Annual Meeting, Hilton Head Island, South Carolina

Morgan, A Dr, Martin K BSc, 2005 *Do electric and magnetic fields cause childhood leukemia?: A review of the scientific evidence"* Children with Leukaemia UK

Moser, M, Schaumberger K, Schernhammer E, Stevens R G, 2006 *Cancer and Rhythm, Cancer Causes Control*, 17:483-487 Springer, Netherlands

Nader, C, 2006 May 13, *Doctors Sceptical about Link*, The Age Newspaper, Fairfax Publications, AUS

Northrup, C Dr, 2001 *The Wisdom of Menopause: The Complete Guide to Creating Physical and Emotional Health and Healing*, Bantam Books, USA

Ogilvie, R, 2006 *Better Breast Health*, Nature & Health Magazine, December 2006/January 2007, Yatta Publishing Group Pty Ltd AUS

Phillips, J B, Deutschlander, M E, 1997 *Magnetoreception in Terrestrial Vertebrates: Implications for Possible Mechanisms of EMF Interaction with Biological Systems* in Richard G Stevens, Bary W Wilson and Larry E Anderson (eds) *The Melatonin Hypothesis: Breast Cancer and Use of Electric Power*, Columbus: Battelle Press, USA

Pierpaoli, W MD PhD, Regelson, W MD 1995 *The Melatonin Miracle*, Simon & Schuster, USA

Portier, C J, 2000 *Decisions about Environmental Health Risks: What are the Key Questions and How Does This Apply to Melatonin?* Low frequency EMF, Visible Light, Melatonin and Cancer International Symposium, May 4-5 2000, University of Cologne, Germany

R K Partnership Ltd, 2007 *Stakeholder Advisory Group on ELF EMFs (SAGE) Precautionary approaches to ELF EMFs First Interim Assessment: Power Lines and Property, Wiring in Homes, and Electrical Equipment in Homes*, UK

Reiter,   R, 1997 *Melatonin Biosynthesis, Regulation, and Effects* in Richard G Stevens, Bary W Wilson and Larry E Anderson (ed) T*he Melatonin Hypothesis: Breast Cancer and Use of Electric Power*, Columbus: Battelle Press, USA

Rogers,   W R, and Reiter, R J and Orr, J L,1997 *Effects of Exposure to 60-Hz EMF on Melatonin in Nonhuman Primates Might Depend on Specific Aspects of Field Exposure* in Richard G Stevens, Bary W Wilson and Larry E Anderson (eds) *The Melatonin Hypothesis: Breast Cancer and Use of Electric Power*, Columbus: Battelle Press, USA

Rose,   P, 2007 *Changes to the Approach to Breast Cancer Screening* The Art of Healing Issue 18 Legit Publications AUS

Sage,   C MA, 2007 *Summary for the Public – The BioInitiative Report: A Rationale for a Biologically – based Public Exposure Standard for Electromagnetic Fields (ELF and RF)*, The BioInitiative Working Group, USA

Schernhammer E, Hankinson, S E, 2005 *Urinary Melatonin Levels and Breast Cancer Risk*, Brief Communications Journal of the National Cancer Institute Vol 97, No. 14 July 20

Shearman,   I, 2001 *Expert Witness Report*, Planning and Environment Court, Brisbane, Queensland, AUS

Slesin,   L PhD, 2002 *Precautionary Limits for EMFs: Why They Are Needed, Microwave News*, Volume XXII No 2 March/April, USA

Slesin,   L PhD, 2007 *Koreans Again Link AM radio to Childhood Leukemia Microwave News*, Volume XXVII No 8 July, USA

Stevens,   R G Dr, 2007, *Meeting Report: the Role of Environmental Lighting an Circadian Disruption in Cancer and Other Diseases* Environ Health Perspect. Sept; 115(9): 1357-62

Stevens,   R G Dr, 2006 *Artificial Lighting in the Industrialized World: Circadian Disruption and Breast Cancer*, Cancer Causes Control May;17(4):501-7

Stevens,   R G Dr, 2005 *Circadian Disruption and Breast Cancer: from Melatonin to Clock Genes*, Epidemiology Mar;16(2):254-8

Stevens,   R G Dr, 2000 *The Melatonin Hypothesis: Circadian Disruption and Breast Cancer* Low frequency EMF, Visible Light, Melatonin and Cancer International Symposium, May 4-5 2000, University of Cologne, Germany

Stevens,   R G, and London, S J, 1997, Breast Cancer in Richard G Stevens, Bary W Wilson and Larry E Anderson (eds) *The Melatonin Hypothesis: Breast Cancer and Use of Electric Power*, Columbus: Battelle Press, USA

Stevens,   R G, Wilson, B W, Anderson, L E (eds) 1997 *The Melatonin Hypothesis: Breast Cancer and Use of Electric Power* Columbus: Battelle Press USA

The Parliament of the Commonwealth of Australia, 2001 *Inquiry into Electromagnetic Radiation* Report of the Senate Environment, Communications, Information Technology and the Arts References Committee, AUS

Verkasalo, P K, Pukkala E, Stevens R G, Ojamo M, Rudanko S L, 2000 *Visual Impairment and Cancer in Finland* Low frequency EMF, Visible Light, Melatonin and Cancer International Symposium, May 4-5 2000, University of Cologne, Germany

Weaver, C, 2007 Cancer *'Cluster' Fear*, The Sunday Telegraph, July 27, News Corporation AUS

Wilson, B W, and Matt, K S, 1997, *Effect of EMF Exposure on the Neuroendocrine System* in Richard G Stevens, Bary W Wilson and Larry E Anderson (eds) *The Melatonin Hypothesis: Breast Cancer and Use of Electric Power*, Columbus: Battelle Press, USA

Wiltschko R, and Wiltschko W, 2006 *Magnetoreception BioEssays* 28:157–168, Wiley Periodicals, Inc. USA

Planning & Environment Court, Brisbane 2001 *Transcripts*, Day Three, AUS

Planning & Environment Court, Brisbane 2001 *Transcripts*, Day Four, AUS

Planning & Environment Court, Brisbane 2001 *Transcripts*, Day Five, AUS

http://jnci.oxfordjournals.org

http://www.ncbi.nlm.nih.gov/sites/entrez

http://www.nzherald.co.nz/section/2/story.cfm?c_id=2&objectid=10463870

www.abc.net.au/austory/content/2007/s1876734.htm, *Million to One* (Part 2) – Transcript

www.aacrjournals.org 2005 Cancer Res; 65(23) December 1

www.bioinitiative.org

www.breastcancerchoices.org/epstein.html

www.brcancerconf.kos.net

www.consumerhealth.org

www.dhs.ca.gov/ehib/emf/RiskEvaluation/ExecSumm.pdf *(Executive Summary of the California EMF Risk Evaluation For Policymakers And the Public, The California Department of Health Services, June 2002).*

www.energyfields.org

www.electric-fields.bris.ac.uk *Powerline report fails to protect the public against health risks*

www.emfacts.com EMFacts Consultancy Latest News and Information Web Log

2007 #795 *Surge in Youth Bipolar Disorder*

2007 #768 *"Freaky" cancer cluster suspected at Sydney hospital*

2007 #767 *Children with Leukaemia Charity's press release on the Cross-Party report*

2007 #766 *Recommendations of the UK Cross-Party Inquiry on Childhood Leukaemia and EMF/EMFs*

2007 #765 *Royal Commission on Environmental Pollution (EMF) on the Agenda*

2007 #764 *WHO recommend precautionary approach for ELF for the first time*

www.iarc.fr/pageroot/PRELEASES/pr16.html 2001 *IARC Finds Limited Evidence that Residential Magnetic Fields Increase Risk of Childhood Leukaemia*, WHO

www.icems.eu

www.leukaemiaconference.org/programme/speakers/day3.asp

www.microwavenews.com
2005 *When Enough is Never Enough: A Reproducible Effect at 2mG-12mG)* November 23
2007 *Weak kHz Electric Fields Kill Tumor Cells*
2007 *News & Comment June 15*

www.neilcherry.com

www.niehs.nih.gov/oc/news/cancerlight.htm 2005 *Artificial Light at Night Stimulates Breast Cancer Growth in Laboratory Mice*

www.news.ninemsn.com.au/sixtyminutes/stories/2001_05_27/story_344.asp
Professor Denis Henshaw on High-Voltage Powerlines

www.powerwatch.org.uk

www.powerwatch.org.uk 2007 *The Sage Report* Powerwatch News 29/4/07

www.powerwatch.org.uk/news/20070429_sage_comments.asp

www.powerwatch.org.uk/reports/20060621_transients_health.pdf

www.pubmed.gov

www.who.int/inf-fs/en/fact263.html 2001 *Electromagnetic Fields and Public Health: Extremely low frequency fields and cancer* WHO

www.int/peh-emf/publications/elf_ehc/en/index.html238 2007, World Health Organisation (WHO) Environmental Health Criteria Monograph on Extremely Low Frequency Fields No. 238

www.wickpedia.org

Consultants

Australia

EMFACTS Consultancy

Don Maisch, of EMFacts Consultancy, Tasmania is available for ELF EMF and RFR EMF testing in buildings. Don Maisch is currently finishing a Doctorate at the University of Wollongong on risk assessment as used in setting radio-frequency standards. Don Maisch advises the Australasian College of Nutritional & Environmental Medicine (www.acnem.org).

The EMFacts website under *Latest News and Information* – Web Log – continually presents updates on the latest research, studies and news relating to EMR.

Contact: **dmaisch@emfacts.com**

Website: **www.emfacts.com**

EMR Australia

EMR Australia has qualified consultants available for ELF EMF and RF EMF testing.

EMR Australia Pty Ltd publishes an independent quarterly newsletter called EMR and HEALTH. This publication contains new studies and articles in relation to electromagnetic radiation – EMR: ELF EMF and RF EMF. EMR Australia's director, Lyn McLean's own experiences with EMR led her to run the EMR Association of Australia and the EMR Alliance of Australia for nine years.

Lyn McLean has published *"Watt's the Buzz"* on understanding and avoiding the risks of electromagnetic radiation, shielding techniques and a more comprehensive list of the studies.

Contact. Phone: **02 9501 2665** (International +61 2 9501 2665).

Website: **www.emraustralia.com.au**

United States of America

Sage EMF Design, Sage Associates in the United States.

Contact: **sage@silcom.com**

Website: **www.silcom.com/~sage/emf/**

Ms Sage participated in The BioInitiative Report.

For more contacts in the USA refer to the website:

www.energyfields.org – Council on Wireless Technology Impacts – Resources section

Canada

EMF Solutions

Website: **www.emfsolutions.ca**

United Kingdom

The Powerwatch Group

Website: **www.powerwatch.org.au**

Other Countries

For all other countries contact a qualified EMF/EMR consultant.

*D*onna Fisher loves a challenge and her very first one came early. At the tender age of 4, like millions of children worldwide she started school. Having stuttered on every letter since she first spoke, reading in class was a real torture. Stuttering can become so serious that it makes a vocational failure of even a talented person but not in Donna's case. Donna overcame her disordered speech over years of labour and today there are only a few letters left for her to overcome. She asserts, with great determination that she will gain fluency. Part of the therapy for gaining fluency and indeed self-confidence is to exercise patience and calmness and this too has gone a long way in finding personal peace and clarity for her.

Although Donna had involved herself in many worthy causes and also successful commercial enterprises it simply wasn't enough to satisfy her drive, energy and restlessness. She likes to be active and in that way she is a "doer". After studying Transpersonal Psychology in 1997 she took the time to attend an intensive workshop on leadership and went on to complete a thesis with special emphasis on the positive role of women in co-creating a better world. That was back in the 1990's.

In 1999, the first Energex letter arrived. Now more than ever Donna's increasing comprehension of owning her own mind combined easily with her patient nature. This led her to study the attributes of the "Warrior Path" and how change can come through peaceful means. Donna volunteered shortly after that for 18 months for a non-profit association dealing with child abuse.

When Donna took on the Energex case she had long learnt that the way forward for personkind is through sharing a reality in a co-creative way and intervening with positive action on humanitarian issues that are particularly important to her.

By claiming and owning one's mind she says humanity can live intelligently through the heart. It is the case, she believes that while a little knowledge can be dangerous, too much knowledge takes away the heart sense.

Born in Australia, Donna lives in sunny Queensland where she and her husband run a successful outlet for a national franchise. Donna is involved in promoting her books and together with a dedicated team chairs the DONNA FISHER SILENT FIELDS Inc. through which she offers practical solutions for "cleaning" electricity. While there is a touch of a crusader in Donna, this energetic person does not invade your privacy but encourages you, albeit with great passion, to examine the issues in the on-going "dirty" electricity debate.